Criminology of Homicidal Poisoning

Michael Farrell

Criminology of Homicidal Poisoning

Offenders, Victims and Detection

Springer

Michael Farrell
Herefordshire
UK

ISBN 978-3-319-59116-2 ISBN 978-3-319-59117-9 (eBook)
DOI 10.1007/978-3-319-59117-9

Library of Congress Control Number: 2017941461

Printed on acid-free paper

This Springer imprint is published by Springer Nature
The registered company is Springer International Publishing AG
The registered company address is: Gewerbestrasse 11, 6330 Cham, Switzerland

Preface

In writing this book, my hope is that it will set out some key components of a criminology of homicidal poisoning that will be useful for readers wishing to have an overview and will provide a structure for further work and development.

I would be happy to receive suggestions to make any future editions of the book more helpful to readers at the following e-mail address: drmjfarrell@bulldog1870.plus.com.

Herefordshire, UK Michael Farrell

Acknowledgements

I am grateful for the support and encouragement offered by the John Trestrail III, toxicologist, New Mexico, US. Federal Bureau of Intelligence Crime Statistics Staff were prompt and helpful in clarifying interpretations of their data. Chief Constable David Thompson and Detective Superintendent Mark Payne, Head of Homicide Investigation, West Midlands Police, UK, kindly took the time to help me with contacts. New York members of staff of Springer were highly professional and supportive throughout especially Editor Katie Chabalko who so quickly saw the potential of the book.

Regarding specific chapters, colleagues were generous with their time and encouragement and I wish to warmly thank the following.

Chapter 3: *Criminal Poisoning in Theory*

Professor Paul Rock, Professor of Criminology, London School of Economics, London, UK

Chapter 4: *Understanding Poisons*

Dean Jones, Senior Forensic Pathology Manager, Forensic Pathology Unit, Home Office Science, UK

Chapter 5: *Poisonous Plants, Animals, Bacteria, and Drugs*

John Trestrail III, Toxicologist, New Mexico, US

Chapter 6: *Elements and 'Other Poisons'*

Professor Paul Dargan, Professor of Clinical Toxicology, Guys Hospital, London, UK

Chapter 7: *Poisoners and Their Characteristics*

Professor Peter Vanezis OBE, Professor of Forensic Medical Sciences, Barts and the London, UK

Chapter 8: *Victims of Poisoning*

Dr. Richard Hough Sr., Department of Criminology and Criminal Justice, University of West Florida, US

Chapter 9: *Detection and Its Avoidance in Poisoning Cases*

Detective Inspector Ian Iliffe, Homicide Investigation, West Midlands Police, UK.

Chapter 10: *Poisoners on Trial*

Lawyer Keith Goodhand, Senior Partner of Goodhand and Forsyth, UK

Again, thank you to all concerned. It hardly needs saying that any shortcomings of the book are entirely my own responsibility.

Contents

About the Author

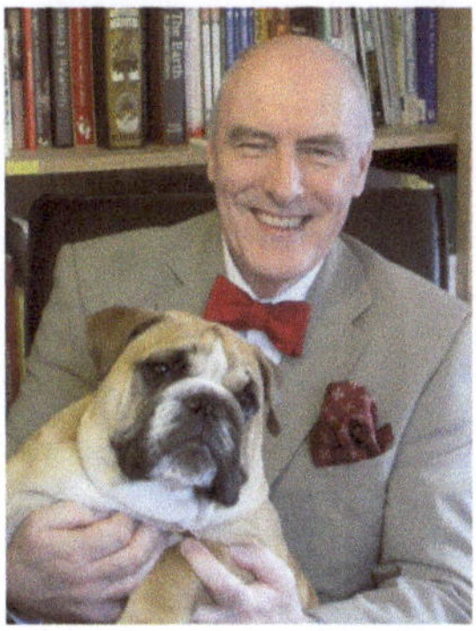

Michael Farrell was educated in the UK. After training as a teacher at Bishop Grosseteste College, Lincoln, and obtaining an honours degree from Nottingham University, he gained an M.A. in Education and Psychology from the Institute of Education, London University. Subsequently, he carried out research for an M.Phil. at the Institute of Psychiatry, London, and for a Ph.D. under the auspices of the Medical Research Council Cognitive Development Unit and London University.

Professionally, Michael Farrell held senior posts in schools and units for people with various mental disorders. He managed a UK-wide psychometric project for City University, London and directed a national initial teacher-training project for the UK Government Department of Education. For over a decade, he led teams inspecting mainstream and special schools and units (boarding, day, hospital, psychiatric). Currently, he works as a private consultant with a range of clients and has lectured or provided consultancy services in various countries including China, Japan, the Seychelles, Australia, Peru, Sweden and the UK.

He has broadcast on the BBC World Service and on UK national radio and has written articles on crime and poisoning in a range of medical, police and legal journals. His many books are translated into European and Asian languages.

Chapter 1
Introduction

Preamble

Throughout these pages walk the men, women and children who have been touched by poisoning. They are perpetrators and victims, their families, friends, neighbours and acquaintances, their lovers and their work colleagues. They are physicians who were called when the victim became ill, pathologists who carried out autopsies and toxicologists who analysed samples from the deceased. They are detectives who investigated the circumstances and lawyers, judges and juries who presented and evaluated the cases in court. It is worth remembering this as we look at issues arising from poisoning because the investigation will often have to be systematic and detached so that it is easy to forget that every 'case' is human tragedy.

Towards a Criminology of Homicidal Poisoning

If we are to consider criminology of homicidal poisoning, several terms need to be clarified quite early in the task. These are criminology itself, homicide and its different types, and the slippery issue of motive.

Criminology

Drawing on sociology, social theory, psychology, history, economics and political science, criminology is concerned with 'social and individual antecedents of crime and with the nature of crime as a social phenomenon'. It involves questions about 'patterns of criminality and their social construction' and the conditions through which they exist whether historical, economic, political or social (Lacey and Zedner 2012, p. 160). In this perspective then, criminology, informed by social sciences, is

M. Farrell, *Criminology of Homicidal Poisoning*,
DOI 10.1007/978-3-319-59117-9_1

concerned with the nature of crime, its antecedents and the conditions that create it as a social phenomenon.

For Rock (2012) criminology is shaped more by its remit than by any theoretical assumptions. It is defined, 'principally by its attachment to an empirical area'. Criminology is 'the study of *crime* that gives unity and order to the enterprise, not adherence to any particular theory or social science' (Ibid., p. 70, italics in original). Alluding to the multidisciplinary nature of criminology, Rock observes that, 'It is in the examination of *crime* that psychologists, statisticians, lawyers, economists, social anthropologists, sociologists, social policy analysts, and psychiatrists meet and call themselves criminologists…' (Ibid., italics in original).

If there is common ground in such perspectives it is that criminology concerns not only crime but its antecedents and context, that there are different theories of crime, and that related to this the subject is multidisciplinary.

Homicide

Regarding homicide, the law in England and Wales for example, reveals certain aspects common to many other countries. Homicide covers the offences of murder and of manslaughter. It also includes other instances of a person causing or being involved in the death of another. In such instances, the general criminal conduct ('actus reus') is the same, that of killing another person, but complex issues arise about causation (Croner 2008, p. 37).

An offence of murder under common law is committed when 'a person unlawfully kills another human being under the Queen's Peace, with malice aforethought' (Croner 2008, p. 37). (A conviction for murder for a person over 18 years old carries a mandatory sentence of life imprisonment). 'Unlawful killing' includes, as well as actively causing another's death, failing to act after creating a situation of danger. In other words, it can involve acts of commission and omission. If there is 'malice aforethought' there is an intention to kill or to cause 'grievous bodily harm' (Ibid., p. 38).

Certain 'special defences' allow for a conviction of manslaughter rather than murder. These are: diminished responsibility (impaired mental responsibility); provocation and a suicide pact (Croner 2008, p. 39). Where such special defences have led the court to a judgement of manslaughter this is classed as 'voluntary manslaughter'. Another category is 'involuntary manslaughter' where a defendant causes the death of another person but is not shown to have the required 'mens rea' for murder. This can involve occasions where the defendant kills another person by, 'an unlawful act which was likely to cause bodily harm; or by gross negligence' (Ibid., p. 41).

Under the *Corporate Manslaughter and Corporate Homicide Act 2007*, an organisation is guilty of an offence if 'the way in which its activities are managed and organised (a) causes a person's death, and (b) amounts to a gross breach of a relevant duty of care owed by the organisation to the deceased' (Sect. 1 of the Act).

Types of Homicide

Types of homicide can be designated in many ways. Perpetrators may be identified such as 'male perpetrated homicide'. Victims may be denoted as with the description, 'infanticide'. Circumstances and location can be specified such as 'domestic homicide'. Yet another way of looking at homicide is to categorise it according to the mode of killing used, for example, 'strangling', 'shooting' or 'stabbing'. As Brookman (2005) notes, one needs to recognise the diversity of homicide. More than this, the various examples (such as 'gang land shootings' and 'the killing of infants') are 'all very different in nature, and the underlying causes are different too' (Ibid., p. 279).

Poison homicide, the topic of this book, specifies the mode of killing. In doing so, it does not exclude further classifications such as the ones already mentioned which might specify the perpetrator, victim or location or other features where these might clarify the picture. Broadly, poisoning seems to be different in nature to some other homicides and may have different underlying explanations.

Motives

One type of explanation for homicide is motive which is essentially an attempt to state why the killing took place. It may not be possible to assign a motive, and even where one is suggested, it may be highly speculative. Also there may be several possible motives that overlap and interact.

We can perhaps describe the general motive for the homicide. This might be for example, financial gain if the victim's life was insured and the perpetrator benefitted from the death. The motive might be to gain sexual freedom to be with a lover, if the victim was a spouse. Other motives might be jealousy, revenge or sadism. If we request more specifically the motive for using poison as the modus operandi, the answers are likely to be different. It may be that the perpetrator calculates that the chances of being caught are less if poison is used instead of for example shooting or stabbing because with poisoning the victim's death might be mistaken for natural causes.

If we extend this line of thinking, it is possible to speak of the motive or motives for various features or events within a homicide. What was the perpetrator's motive for disposing of the body of a victim whom they have poisoned rather than trying to convey that death was from natural causes? What was the motive for choosing a legitimately prescribed medication which the individual was already taking in order to administer a poison overdose? Each of these queries raises other questions and issues.

When the supposed traits of poisoners are discussed, there can sometimes be an overlap with motive. Some traits are distinctive enough. For example, it may be suggested that poisoners tend to be 'calculating'. It is clear that being calculating is not a motive for poison homicide but that it is quality that might help in its execution. However a trait of 'avariciousness' may be suggested (Trestrail 2007, pp. 50–52). This can also be closely related to a motive of greed perhaps for financial gain. The perpetrator killed from a motive of financial gain, being driven by that motive because they were avaricious.

If motive is taken to be a subjective matter, demonstrating motive is likely to involve examples of behaviour that indicate the driving force. If a motive is jealousy, this could be shown where the perpetrator had expressed jealous sentiments to others or to the victim verbally or perhaps in letters. The credibility of a motive of financial gain might be shown (depending on the context) where the perpetrator is demonstrated to care a great deal about money or can be shown to be in great need of money.

In brief, when discussing motive one often uses a broad category such as 'jealousy' or 'financial gain' which can be helpful to describe the overall picture. However, sometimes it may be clearer to specify to what action the term 'motive' applies. This can help us to remember that there may be different motives for different aspects of the sequence of events that are gathered together under the term 'homicide'. Also there can be an overlap with supposed traits where the motive can be a subjective explanation (avarice) of an external feature (financial gain). Attempting to demonstrate motive may involve pointing to examples of what the perpetrator has said or done in different contexts.

Aims of the Book

Using cases of homicidal poisoning, this book sets out the parameters of what might constitute a criminology of homicidal poisonings by:

- Reviewing theories of crime and homicide in relation to poison murder
- Explaining the nature and variety of poisons used in homicidal cases
- Exploring the characteristics of poisoners and their victims in the context of poisoning homicide
- Discussing aspects of detecting poison homicide, and how perpetrators try to avoid detection
- Looking at some issues arising when poisoners are brought to trial.

Scope of the Book

It has been said that poisoning is a comparatively rare form of homicide arising in 3–6% of known homicide cases (Adelson 1974). However, an analysis of Uniform Crime Reports 1980s for the US by Westveer, Trestrail and Pinizzotto (1996) indicated that the unknown offender rate for poisoning cases was 20–30 times higher than that for other homicides. Had serial poisoner Dr. Harold Shipman [81] not been arrested after attempting to forge a patient's Will, around 250 murders of his patients carried out over decades would have likely gone undetected (The square brackets after a poisoner's name refer to the number order in which they are listed in the glossary of this book). As the resulting public enquiry into Shipman's crimes made clear, the public cannot be complaisant that similar activities are going undetected in the future (Shipman Enquiry 2002–2005).

This book examines homicidal poisonings in the modern era with the emphasis on individuals poisoning other individuals. I also touch on rare instances where more than one person carried out the killing or where a small group of people are simultaneously poisoned by an individual. Focusing on the modern era allows us to infer implications for contemporary understanding of poisons, poisoners, detection and prosecution. Where cases are mentioned, throughout the book, they are almost invariably those were a person or persons have been convicted of murder. While most cases are from North America or the United Kingdom, there are examples from Europe (France, Germany, Austria, Switzerland, Norway); Australia; South Africa, Japan, India, China and Indonesia. Because the cases raise important issues, and show the way that poisoners operate, many have been written about in books or articles and entries on internet sites. This chronological, geographical and well-documented range of cases I believe allows them to be used to illustrate points about poisoners and their victims and other factors that are relevant to understanding homicidal poisonings.

Having a focus as just described means that certain types of cases are **not** discussed. These are: 'not proven' cases under the Scottish legal system (Farrell 1989a, 1992b); acquittals either at the one and only trial (Farrell 1994a, 1994c) or at subsequent retrials (Farrell 1992c, 1996); cases where the accused was found guilty but later pardoned (Farrell 1993b); 'mysteries', where it is evident that poisoning has occurred but there is insufficient evidence to charge an individual (Farrell 1993a, b); poisoning as judicial killing (Farrell 1994b); mass poisonings including in wartime; corporate homicide and mass suicide pacts. In February 2017 Kim Jong-nam the half-brother of the North Korean leader Kim Jong-un was apparently assassinated at Kuala Lumpur airport by an assailant wiping a chemical liquid over the victim's face (Reuters and Daily Telegraph 2017). Such assassinations certainly demonstrate that poisoning is still a current issue but are not covered in the present book as the motivations and implications appear to be different to what might be considered more conventional poisonings. Also, cases where the accused died before trail (Farrell 1992a) are not generally discussed although there are a few exceptions to this.

Proposed Readers

Core readers of the book are likely to be: students of criminology (classes dealing with criminal psychology, and murder investigation); criminal justice professionals: attorneys, homicide detectives, forensic pathologists, forensic and clinical toxicologists and other forensic investigators; and more widely, others who are interested in poisons and poisoners and the detection of poisoning. Disciplines of relevance include: criminology, law and policing, toxicology and forensic science, history of crime and detection, criminal psychology and related areas.

An Indication of Subsequent Chapters

For the detailed structure of each chapter, please consult the contents list. In this section, I briefly give a flavour of each chapter.

The chapter on 'Instructive poisoning cases' covers recent cases mainly from the US and UK. From the United States, these are the cases of Paul Marshall Curry [95], Kristin Rossum [82], and Julia Lynn Turner [88]. United Kingdom cases are those of Roger and David Cooper [99], Dr. Harold Shipman [81], and Lakvir Singh [93]. From Indonesia, we consider the poisoning by Jessica Wongso [100]. For each we look at the case in outline then at points of special interest.

In Chap. 3, on 'Criminal poisoning in theory' we look at theories and explanations of crime in general and especially of homicide in the broad sense and then consider the extent to which these apply to poisoning homicide. Biological, psychological and sociological theories are examined.

Chapter 4, 'Understanding Poisons' presents an overview of the nature of poisons. We consider how poisons are defined and classified, how their characteristics are described, and what features less detectable poisons possess. We touch on differences between poison homicides and other homicides. Next we look at the administration, action and fatal doses of poisons. Acute and chronic poisoning is discussed. Finally, we consider antidotes and treatment for poisoning, and possible trends in poisoning

More specifically, the next two chapters look at different poisons used in homicides. In Chap. 5, these are plant poisons such as opium and morphine, animal poisons, for example, cantharides, bacterial poisons like typhoid and drugs such as succinylcholine chloride. Chapter 6 considers elements, their compounds and derivatives for example arsenic and thallium, and 'other poisons', for example, carbon monoxide and antifreeze.

Chapter 7 looks at poisoners and their characteristics and at attempts to identify such characteristics and typologies of poisoners. We discuss gender, age and race in relation to homicide in general and for poison homicide in particular. For each of these factors, illustrative poison cases are outlined. The occupation/social background of poisoners is examined. Multiple poison homicides are also discussed. Acute and chronic poisoning is considered.

In Chap. 8, we discuss the victims of poisoning. Again we look at gender, age, race and occupation for homicide in general and for poison homicide. We examine relationships between offender and victim such as spouse and medic-patient.

Location of the homicide is discussed. We consider why a victim is chosen and how events unfolded.

In looking at detection and its avoidance in poisoning cases (Chap. 9), we consider such issues as apparent cause of death and physical evidence of poisoning; exhumation and autopsy, forensic testing, motives, opportunity and other matters each time looking at how the poisoner might evade detection.

Chapter 10 discusses 'poisoners on trial' and includes what needs to be proved in poison trials and what defences and explanations are offered. As well, we look at the character of the perpetrator, the role and credibility of witnesses technical evidence circumstantial evidence and motive.

A conclusion chapter brings together various themes, while a glossary (described below) presents over a hundred poison cases.

Features of the Book

In style, I have tried to be direct and to avoid jargon and technical terms and, where such terms are necessarily used, to explain them. Chapter structure is intended to aid the assimilation of the information in it, each having an introduction, structured headings and subheadings, a conclusion, suggested activities to encourage reflection and discussion, texts for further reading and chapter references.

The glossary gives key facts on poison cases in broadly chronological sequence according to the year when the perpetrator was sentenced. Where in the body of the book a particular case is mentioned, this is identified by a number in square brackets which relates to the glossary. For example, the recent case of Jessica Wongso from Indonesian convicted of poisoning her friend with cyanide is designated as '[100]'. The glossary outlines just over 100 poisonings from the mid-nineteenth century to the present day including examples of a wide variety of poisons from different parts of the world. Where a poisoner was suspected of other deaths, while usually noting this, I have taken a conservative view and assumed only that they are demonstrably guilty only of the crimes for which they were convicted. There are exceptions to this such as Dr. Harold Shipman, where a public enquiry was held which over several years gathered evidence that pointed to the number of murders that he had perpetrated. Where the sources are press reports, I have distilled from several what appears to be a reliable and consistent account of the crime, but have usually given a single source as an example of the coverage.

The book includes references to other books, chapters, articles, legal and public enquiry documents and internet resources. I have tried to balance good sources with availability so that for many references, readers will be able to access the relevant documents through libraries, book stores, the Internet and elsewhere.

Moving on

We have defined criminology and homicide and outlined different We have briefly discussed the nature of motive. Aims of the book were listed and the scope of the book was explained as covering poison homicide in the modern era. Proposed readers were identified. An indication of what the various chapters of the text cover was provided to supplement the structured contents outline. The main features of the book were touched on. Having set the scene, we can now move on to look at several poisoning cases and the issues that arise which is the subject of the next chapter.

References

Adelson, L. (1974) Murder by poison. In C. Charles (Ed.), *The pathology of homicide.* IL: Springfield.

Brookman, F. (2005). *Understanding homicide.* London and Los Angeles: Sage.

Corporate Manslaughter and Corporate Homicide Act 2007 Chapter 19.

Croner, P. (2008) *Blackstone's police manual 2009: Volume 1—Crime* (11th ed.). Oxford and New York: Oxford University Press.

Farrell, M. (1989a). Arsenic poisoning: The role of legal controls. *Solicitors Journal, 133*(35), 1101–1102.

Farrell, M. (1992a). Poison cases in which the accused died before trial or verdict. *Justice of the Peace, 156*(6), 94–95.

Farrell, M. (1992b) Not proven poison cases. *The Criminologist, 16*(2), 29–31.

Farrell, M. (1992c, March 19) Keep the phial open. *Solicitors Journal, 136*(48), 1266–1267.

Farrell, M. (1993a) What's your poison? *Solicitors Journal.* March 19, 1993, p. 254.

Farrell, M. (1993b) 'Poison Cases Pardoned After Trial' *Justice of the Peace* 157, 17, 269–270.

Farrell, M. (1993c). Poison mysteries. *The Criminologist, 17*(1), 12–14.

Farrell, M. (1994a). Poison acquittals at the first and only trial. *Justice of the Peace, 158*(21), 339–341.

Farrell, M. (1994b). Execution by poison gas and lethal injection. *The Criminologist, 18*(4), 201–204.

Farrell, M. (1994c). Adelaide bartlett and the pimlico mystery. *British Medical Journal, 6970* (308), 1720–1723.

Farrell, M. (1996). Poison cases—Acquittals at re-trial. *The Criminologist, 20*(4), 236–239.

Fifth Report. (2004, December). *Safeguarding patients: Lessons from the part—Proposals for the future.*

First Report. (2002, July). *Volume 1—Death disguised; Volume 2—Decisions Todmorden; Volumes 3–6—Decisions Hyde.*

Fourth Report. (2004, July). *The regulation of controlled drugs in the community.*

Lacey, N., & Zedner, L. (2012). Legal constructions of crime. In M. Maguire, R. Morgan, & R. Reiner (Eds.), *The Oxford handbook of criminology* (5th ed.). Oxford: Oxford University Press.

Reuters and Daily Telegraph. (2017, February). Kim Jong-nam murder: Japanese network releases CCTV footage of assassination of North Korean leader's half-brother.

Rock, P. (2012). Sociological theories of crime. In M. Maguire, R. Morgan, & R. Reiner. (2012). *The Oxford handbook of criminology* (5th ed., pp. 39–80).Oxford: Oxford University Press.

Second Report. (2003, July). *The police investigation of March 1998.* Cm 5853.

Sixth Report. (2005, January). *Shipman: The final report.*

The Shipman Inquiry http://webarchive.nationalarchives.gov.uk/20090808154959/http://www.the-shipman-inquiry.org.uk/fr_page.asp

Third Report. (2003, July). *Death certification and the investigation of deaths by coroners.*

Trestrail, J. H. (2007). *Criminal poisoning: Investigational guide for law enforcement, toxicologists, forensic scientists and attorneys* (2nd ed.). Totowa, NJ, Humana Press.

Westveer, A. E., Trestrail, J. H., & Pinizotto, J. (1996). Homicidal poisonings in the United States —An analysis of the uniform crime reports from 1980 through 1989. *American Journal of Forensic Medicine and Pathology, 17*(4), 282–288.

Chapter 2
Instructive Poison Cases

Introduction

In this chapter, we will look at several cases and, for each, identify points of particular relevance with reference to perpetrators: Roger and David Cooper [99], Paul Marshall Curry [95], Harold Shipman [81], Lynn Turner [88], Lakhvir Singh [93], Kristin Rossum [82] and Jessica Wongso [100].

Roger and David Cooper, UK

The Case

On Christmas Eve 2014, Costco boss Roger Cooper and his brother David Cooper, a doorman, of Leicester, England conspired to poison Sameena Imam, Roger's lover and co-worker. To prevent Sameena exposing their 2-year affair, Roger spent a month plotting to kill her, buying poisonous metals and identifying a location in which to bury the body. David helped Roger to kill the victim and he disposed of the body.

In late November 2014, Sameena Imam booked a stay at the Malmaison Hotel, Birmingham for herself and Roger for December 24 and 25. She was led to believe that Roger intended to leave his long-term partner for a future with her, starting with a shared Christmas at the Birmingham hotel.

On Christmas Eve, at around 4 p.m., Roger left the Costco store in Coventry (where he and Sameena were both working) ahead of Sameena and they drove off in their separate cars. Later meeting up nearby, the couple left Sameena's car on a side road. Sameena transferred her hotel luggage into Roger's car before the pair headed to David Cooper's Leicester address for what she thought was a brief Christmas visit. At the house, the brothers overpowered her on a settee, killing her

M. Farrell, *Criminology of Homicidal Poisoning*,
DOI 10.1007/978-3-319-59117-9_2

by holding a tea towel doused in chloroform over her mouth. David later buried the body at his allotment (a plot of land used for non-commercial gardening).

On Boxing Day, David drove from his Leicester home, picked up Sameena's car in Coventry, and drove it back to his address. Next day, he drove the car to Luton and abandoned it in a side street, next taking a taxi to Luton rail station and travelling back to Leicester. On December 29, he collected a hire car from Coventry and travelled to Luton once more where he moved Sameena's car again and used cleaning agent to wipe away any trace of fingerprints and DNA.

Sameena had been reported missing when she failed to join her family in Essex as planned for Boxing Day and a police enquiry was initiated. Police interviewed Roger as a significant witness on January 1 and 2. David was questioned as a witness on January 4. The brothers were arrested on 7 January 2015 on suspicion of murder and on January 9 were charged, despite Sameena's body still not having been found.

Initially, David made a partial admission to having pressed a chloroform-soaked tea towel over Sameena's mouth but claimed that her death had been accidental. Later still in court he stated that he had found Ms Imam's body after being asked to move a car. Roger Copper told police that he last saw the victim when she left the Costco store at about 4 p.m. on December 24.

A female friend of David's contacted police on January 11 to report that David had given her a set of keys before being arrested. They were for his Leicester allotment. Later that day, officers visited the allotment and excavations by forensic specialists began the following day. Sameena's body was found in a grave 5 days later and subsequently an autopsy was carried out. Guided by Roger Cooper's confession, indications of possible poisoning by chloroform were found. Also, toxicological tests requested for chloroform established that the victim had been poisoned by the substance. It appeared that a combination of metallic elements, including antimony, cadmium, tin, mercury and arsenic had also been administered to Sameena Imam in a liquid.

At the trial at Birmingham, computer printouts of David Cooper's eBay purchase history for December 8 showed that he bought chloroform. While admitting making the purchase, he claimed that it had never arrived. Evidence was presented of mobile phone messages linked to David showing that the brothers had made a previous attempt on Ms Imam's life on 11 December which may have been aborted because she arrived at the arranged meeting place too conspicuously. Telephone evidence also supported Roger and Sameena's joint arrival at around 5 p.m. in Leicester where it is believed that the victim was very soon killed. At 6.25 p.m. Roger began his return journey to Coventry leaving David to dispose of the body. Evidence showed that when Roger got to Coventry he used Sameena's mobile phone to send himself a text message to suggest that she was still alive and well.

Automatic number plate recognition hits showed the vehicles that the brothers had used travelling between Coventry and Leicester. A bottle of Bellini drink shown to have been bought in Coventry by Ms Imam on Christmas Eve was also found in the refrigerator at David's home.

Roger Cooper's motive appeared to be to conceal the affair with Sameena. She believed that their relationship would now be open, and widely known. He feared that this would lose him his job at Costco which forbids intimate relationships within the management structure, and jeopardise the long-term relationship with his partner. But it is unclear why his brother agreed to help to kill someone whom he had only briefly met. Found guilty at Birmingham Crown Court, the brothers were each sentenced to 30 years imprisonment.

Points of Special Interest

Poisoning is normally used where the deceased's body is left in situ. Usually, the intention is that murder will not be detected because death might appear to be from natural causes or suicide for example. In this case, the body was disposed of with the hoped that it would not be found. Chloroform was apparently used to silently subdue the victim so that no sounds of a struggle would be heard.

Another feature was the careful planning involved by the perpetrators to suggest that the deceased was still alive when she was not, to lay false trails about the brothers' movements, and to try to remove any detrimental traces from the deceased's car. However, thorough investigation enabled the prosecution to present evidence of telephone contacts, indications of the journeys taken, shop receipts and records of eBay transactions all building up an incriminating picture. Changing accounts provided by David, and the evidence contradicting Roger's version of events provided the jury with further evidence to find the pair guilty.

Relatively few examples are available of a person being poisoned and then the body being disposed of. Dr. Crippen [35] poisoned his wife then buried the body in the cellar of his house claiming that she had left him. Arthur Deveureux [31] disposed of the bodies of his wife and twin sons whom he poisoned. Also, French physician Dr. Marcel Petiot [55] killed potential escapees from Nazi occupied France with cyanide injections before burning the bodies.

Paul Marshall Curry, US

The Case

At his trial in 2014, Paul Marshall Curry then 58 years old and from Salina, Kansas, was convicted of the murder of his third wife perpetrated over 20 years earlier. It was a prime example of a cold case being successfully revisited by investigators.

Paul Curry met Linda in 1989 while both worked at the San Onofre nuclear power plant in northern San Diego County, California. Although 13 years older, she would become his third wife. They lived in San Clemente where within a year of marriage Curry began poisoning his wife. In 1993 Linda Curry was hospitalised several times suffering unexplained vomiting, headaches and bloody diarrhoea. In one such visit, hospital staff discovered lidocaine in Linda Curry's intravenous (IV) bag and suspected tampering. An overdose of lidocaine, a tissue numbing medication, can be fatal, and the couple were questioned. Linda told investigators in a recorded interview that the only person of whom she could think who might harm her was her husband, and the only motive she could contemplate was money. She did not want to believe this was so. Paul Curry claimed that he had nothing to gain from his wife's death.

From 1993 through to mid-1994, Curry then a nuclear power plant engineer secretly administered his wife small doses of nicotine. On 9 June 1994, Curry gave Linda sleeping pills before injecting a final fatal dose of nicotine behind her ear. Calling the 911 emergency services, Curry reported that he had found his wife in bed and not breathing. Orange County emergency services got Linda Curry to hospital where she died a few hours later.

It was only a day after the funeral was held that Curry began trying to collect life insurance benefits, over a period claiming $547,000. Even at the time, police suspected Curry of murder. Linda had been a non-smoker, so lethal amounts of nicotine in her system were difficult to explain. However, investigators lacked sufficient evidence to press charges.

Curry moved to North Las Vegas, Nevada where he worked as a senior plans examiner. In the meantime, investigators uncovered fresh evidence shortening the time that it would have taken Curry to administer the lethal nicotine injection, a previous stumbling block. In March 2010, he relocated to Kansas after being hired by the city of Salina and was arrested the same year by which time he had a new job as chief county building inspector.

Sent for trial at Santa Ana, Orange County, California, Curry appeared before Judge Patrick Donahue. Prosecutor Ebrahim Baytieh pointed out Curry's financial gain from Linda's insurance, suggesting that he had an, 'insatiable appetite for money'. A former wife Leslie, who had been married to Curry before he met Linda, testified that in the last year of their marriage she was constantly ill. Curry suggested that they both apply for life insurance. They did so but while his application was accepted, hers was rejected. Soon after, the couple separated and Leslie moved back to Las Vegas where her family lived. Once apart from her husband, her health recovered.

Defence attorney Lisa Kopelman told jurors that Curry was a loving husband who nursed his chronically sick wife. Arguing that Linda was often ill with digestive ailments, the lawyer suggested that she may have taken nicotine as a treatment for irritable bowel syndrome. The large amount found in her system may have being owing to a self-administered nicotine enema used as a holistic treatment. Indeed, Linda Curry had had illnesses for several years before she married. Also it was argued there was little direct evidence pointing to Curry's guilt.

In the event, the jury found Curry guilty of 'first-degree murder, with special circumstances for poisoning and murder for financial gain'. Curry was sentenced to life imprisonment without parole.

Points of Special Interest

Among points raised by the Curry case are that evidence can emerge after a long period and prosecutions can still be secured, but even for a 'cold case' this was a lengthy interim. Defence lawyers had put forward a motion that Paul Curry was denied his right to due process because of the delayed prosecution but that was rejected.

Linda Curry not being a smoker and yet nicotine being found in her system had remained suspicious. Her view that her husband could be the only one harming her that she had expressed at the hospital in 1993 had been recorded and was played to the court. Furthermore, the time frame in which Curry could be assumed to have given the lethal dose was originally thought to make it difficult to claim that he had been the killer. But later findings allowed this time scale to be shortened.

Circumstantial evidence that a former wife Leslie may have also been given poisoned by Curry added to the picture of potential guilt. Claiming that the motive was greed was conversant with Curry's precipitate claiming of insurance money, and supported the testimony that a similar pattern may have been attempted with another former spouse. The prosecution argument that poisoning was deliberate was met by the defence suggestion that the substance could have been taken medicinally by the deceased.

Dr. Harold Shipman, UK

The Case

Dr. Harold Shipman (1946–2004) was the UKs most prolific serial killer. In June 1963 when Harold was aged 17 years, his mother died of lung cancer. While still attending school, he looked after her and witnessed the doctor administering morphine to ease pain. Three years later, aged 19, he married Primrose Oxtoby, a 17 year old from North Yorkshire, pregnant with his child. Their marriage lasted throughout Shipman's life.

Accepted into medical school at the University of Leeds in 1965, Shipman graduated 5 years later, aged 25 years. He was appointed preregistration House Officer at Pontefract General Infirmary and a year later was fully registered as a doctor by the General Medical Council. Shipman spent 3 years as a Senior House Officer and gained higher diplomas. Entering general practice in 1974, he was appointed to the Abraham Ormerod Medical Practice at Todmorden, where after a probationary period, he became a junior partner. Shipman stayed until September 1979 when his colleagues discovered that he had been dishonestly obtaining controlled drugs (pethidine) for his own use. In 1979, he pleaded guilty in court to drugs charges, and the General Medical Council took no action against him.

The following year, he became a General Practitioner at the Donneybrook practice in Hyde, a small industrial town south west of Manchester, admitting his criminal record at the appointment interview. Having left the Donneybrook practice in January 1992, Shipman began working as a sole practitioner in the same building. In October, he moved to the Market Street surgery nearby, again as a sole practitioner. For the great majority of those who knew him, he was a well-liked and respected doctor in the community.

In March 1998, some people in Hyde expressed concern at the number of Shipman's elderly patients who were dying in similar circumstances. Dr. Linda Reynolds, from the nearby Brooke Practice, alerted the South Manchester Coroner, John Pollard, to concerns about the number of Shipman's patients who were dying and the circumstances. Following a request from the Coroner, Greater Manchester Police conducted a confidential investigation. It was conducted by Detective Inspector (DI) David Smith under the supervision of Chief Superintendent (CS) David Sykes. DI Smith concluded that there was no substance in Dr. Reynolds' concerns, ending the investigation on 17 April 1998 after which Shipman killed three more patients before being arrested.

In 1998 a former mayor of Hyde, Kathleen Grundy, aged 81, died at home, having been a patient of Dr. Shipman. Her daughter, Angela Woodruff a solicitor, was puzzled by aspects of her mother's death, but it was duly registered. She was then surprised to find that her mother's Will which she knew had left her estate to near relatives had been changed in favour of Dr. Shipman shortly before Kathleen's death. Angela Woodruff reported her suspicions to the police. Greater Manchester Police started to investigate the death of Kathleen Grundy, searching Shipman's surgery and his home. Kathleen's body was exhumed and toxicology tests showed the presence of unexpectedly high levels of morphine in tissue samples. Police looked into 19 deaths that had been brought to light by the investigation in March and further exhumations were carried out showing the presence of morphine in the bodies. When Shipman's computerised medical records were examined, it was evident that they had been changed to make it appear that patients had had long established illnesses leading to their death so that the real cause of death by morphine was unsuspected. Shipman was arrested and charged with murder.

In 1999, Shipman was tried at Preston Crown Court on 15 counts of murder and the forging of the Kathleen Grundy's Will, pleading 'not guilty' to all charges. Found guilty on all counts, he was given a prison term of 15 life sentences and 4 years for forgery. The Director of Public Prosecutions stated that no further criminal proceedings would be started, it being impossible for Shipman to have a fair trial.

Before the trial and following it, police investigated many deaths of Shipman's patients where there was evidence that Shipman was responsible. Those deaths were reported to the South Manchester Coroner, who, between August 2000 and April 2001, conducted inquests into 27 deaths of Shipman's patients, recording verdicts of unlawful killing in 25 and open verdicts in 2. In May 2001, the Coroner opened inquests into a further 232 deaths, then immediately adjourned them, pending publication of the findings of a public Inquiry.

The enquiry established in 2001 and chaired by Dame Janet Smith produced a series of reports. Report 1 found that Shipman killed 215 of his patients, the first, Mrs. Eva Lyons, in March 1975, when Shipman was practising in Todmorden, and the last, Mrs. Kathleen Grundy, in June 1998. (Report 1, Vol 1 summary para15). By the time of the sixth and final report, the estimate was that Shipman started killing earlier (in 1971) and murdered about 250 patients between 1971 and 1998, of whom the inquiry was able positively to identify 218. The usual method of killing was administering a lethal dose of an opiate (usually diamorphine). Shipman committed suicide in Wakefield Prison on 13 January 2004.

Points of Special Interest

Probably the foremost question in this case is how the crimes could go undetected for so long. As well as subverting the procedures for death certification, Shipman combined the high respect in which he was held by many patients with the harsh dismissal of concerns of relatives to prevent suspicion. When concerns were eventually raised with authorities, the police enquiry was hampered by the lack of experience of officers directly involved, and a tendency on behalf of the advising doctor to believe that there was nothing wrong.

The use of morphine-based drugs to kill was disguised by various features. Shipman as a physician was allowed to use the drugs. He was in a position to determine the cause of death. Also, especially where elderly or ill patients were involved, the deaths were to varying degrees 'expected'. Evidence presented at the trial included autopsy and other toxicological evidence, computer medical records indicating tampering and the forged Will.

Julia Lynn Turner, US

The Case

Born in 1968, by her early twenties, Lynn Womack (as she was called before marriage) worked as a 911 dispatcher for Cobb County, Georgia. There she met local police officer Glenn Turner whom she married in 1992. Lynn Turner left her job and despite Glenn working an extra job at a gas station, his income was still insufficient to support his wife's lavish spending. Their relationship deteriorated and Lynn began a secret affair with Randy Thompson, a Forsyth County firefighter.

In 1995, Glenn started plans to move out and file for a divorce but fell ill. He visited the emergency room of Kennestone Hospital in March 1995 complaining of symptoms that seemed to suggest influenza. After being given intravenous fluids and medication, he returned their Marietta home. Lynn's account was that on returning home, Glenn took a turn for the worse. Waking after midnight, he had hallucinations and went down to the basement where he tried to drink gasoline. Lynn helped him back upstairs and the next morning he seemed to be feeling better. Lynn went out to do some errands and when she returned found Glenn dead. Cause of death was put down to natural causes owing to an irregular heartbeat. Lynn moved in with Randy and collected substantial life insurance on her husband's death.

Lynn and Randy bought a house and had two children Blake and Amber, but by 2000 they were having relationship problems and Randy moved out into an apartment. On 21 January 2001, Randy was feeling ill and visited the emergency room with symptoms of vomiting and stomach ache. He was treated and released the same day. The following day however, the 32 year old was found dead in his apartment. Lynn again collected money resulting from her boyfriend's death which was caused by irregular heartbeat.

Tests found ethylene glycol based antifreeze in Thompson's blood. Now Glenn Turner's body was exhumed and evidence of antifreeze poisoning was found in his kidneys. Crime scene photographs from Glenn's death were examined and one was found to show the garage were antifreeze could be seen. Late in 2001, Lynn was arrested for the murder of Glenn Turner.

Put on trial in 2004, she was found guilty. Although she was not charged with the murder of Randy Thompson's death at that time, the prosecution was allowed to refer to evidence of the similarities between the two deaths.

Vince Turley, a former insurance agent, stated that before Glenn and Lynn were married and she was his fiancée, she requested that Glenn made her the beneficiary should he die. Glenn complied in September 1993. Animal shelter worker, Samantha Gilleland stated that Lynn Turner has made several visits to the shelter and, discussing stray cats, had learned that antifreeze would poison them. The emergency room physician Dr. Donald Freeman who treated Glenn Turner the day before he died testified that symptoms did not suggest a single large ingestion of ethylene glycol and that Glenn Turner may have ingested smaller amounts of the poison over a period of several days.

Dr. Brian Frist, the Cobb County medical examiner, performed the autopsy on Glenn Turner in 1995 giving cause of death as heart failure. Microscopically, he did though find calcium oxalate crystals in Glenn Turner's tissue. It was only when he heard of the death of Randy Thompson that he reconsidered the presence of the crystals and the findings and ordered Turner's body to be exhumed. Realising with hindsight the significance of the findings he stated his belief that 'they are the result of ethylene glycol toxicity'. Dr. Kris Sperry the Chief Medical Examiner at the Georgia Bureau of Investigation, testified that Randy Thomson may have first consumed antifreeze up to 2 days before we visited the emergency room on 20 January 2001. He likely ingested more antifreeze later given the levels of ethylene glycol found in his body after death. Crime laboratory analyst Chris Tilson of the Georgia Bureau of Investigation stated that lethal levels of ethylene glycol were not detected straight away in Randy Thompson's body because he had made a 'mathematical calculation error' in the analysis. When a medical examiner found calcium oxalate crystals in Thompson's kidneys (indicative of ethylene glycol poisoning) further test were conducted.

For the defence, Helen Gregory, Lynn Turner's mother testified that on the day of Glenn Turner's death, Lynn was, 'crying hysterically'. She stated that Lynn's apparent coldness at the funerals of her husband and common law husband was because she does not openly show 'her feelings and emotions'. Also for the defence, toxicologist Dr. Robert Palmer raised the question of whether the calcium oxalate crystals found where Turner's body was exhumed could be from embalming fluids, flowers or other materials decomposing inside the coffin. He stated that the crystals found in Glenn Turner's kidneys would have been expected to be detected in other bodily organs too.

In 2007, Lynn Turner was tried and convicted for the murder of Randy Thompson, receiving a sentence of life imprisonment without parole. On August 2010, aged 42 years old, Lynn Turner was found dead in a cell shared with several other inmates at Metro State Prison. She may have committed suicide by accumulating medication for raised blood pressure and taking a lethal overdose.

Points of Special Interest

This is an example of a case where the perpetrator had committed murder once and gone undetected and was only caught when she tried the same modus operandi a second time. It is worth reflecting on such cases when one considers poisoning statistics, as had Lynn Turner not tried a second killing it is unlikely that she would have come to police attention.

While methanol antifreeze ('methyl alcohol') is colourless, smells slightly of alcohol and is soluble in water, it has a burning taste making it detectable in bland foods. However, ethylene glycol antifreeze (1,2 ethanol) used by Lynn Turner is odourless and highly soluble in water but sweet tasting making it unlikely to be detected in food.

While it seems plain that Lynn Turner's broad motive in both murders was financial gain the timing is interesting. The timing of her first husband's murder prevented his filing for divorce and that of her boyfriend was perpetrated before their deteriorating relationship jeopardised the prospect of financial gain.

Lakvir Singh, UK

The Case

Complicated relationships within several families emerged in the case of Lakvir Singh. Following the failure of his first marriage Lakhvinder 'Lucky' Cheema and

Lakvir Singh had been clandestine lovers. The relationship started when Cheema, a cleaner, moved into his family's home in Southall, West London. Singh then aged 20 was caught in a loveless marriage and was attracted to the new tenant. Later Cheema bought his own home in Feltham, Middlesex and the relationship continued. Singh became pregnant twice over this period but each time had an abortion, Cheema being afraid of the shame that their affair would bring if it were found out.

So Singh visited Cheema's house every day to clean, cook and do laundry for 16 years until October 2008. At that date, Lakvir Singh was 45, married to Aunkar Singh aged 57 and had three children. Cheema was 39. Cheema was introduced to Gurjeet Choongh an illegal immigrant aged 21 to whom he became engaged. Determined to marry his fiancé, Cheema broke off the long affair with Singh.

Singh sent text messages to her lover urging him to end the engagement, calling him a 'bastard' and saying that her heart was broken. Outside the house, after spotting Cheema in bed with his fiancé, she peered through the window and threatened to burn down his house. Cheema refused to end the relationship with the younger woman. Singh then took a trip to India and in December returned with a quantity of aconite with which to poison her former lover.

At the time of the murder, Singh's husband who had cancer was abroad receiving treatment. On 27 January 2009, Lakvir Singh of Southall, West London, slipped into Cheema's home in Feltham, Middlesex, England and sprinkled the poison into curry stored in a plastic container in the refrigerator. She knew that the couple were planning to eat the curry that same evening. Choongh microwaved the leftover curry and then served the two of them at the dining table.

Cheema and his fiancée ate the curry while discussing plans for their wedding which was scheduled to take place a few weeks later on Valentine's Day. Cheema had second helpings. Soon after the meal Cheema became ill and made an emergency 999 call in which he stated that his ex-girlfriend had poisoned him. Cheema also telephoned his sister asking her to come round to the house. He began to vomit, his face became numb and he lost his sight and the use of his limbs. Gurjeet Choongh was also gravely ill with similar symptoms. Cheema's sister Mrs. Khalon and her two sons arrived at the house. Cheema's nephews Gurinder and Surinder Singh helped Cheema into a car to go to hospital. The ill couple were taken to the West Middlesex Hospital. Within an hour of admission, Cheema died in great pain. Gurjeet Choongh having eaten less of the meal appears to have had the better chance of survival. In any event, she was placed in an induced coma to stabilise her heart beat and recovered.

The trial took place at the Old Bailey in 2010. Prosecution argued that Singh has killed Cheema and attempted to kill Choongh from revenge. The defence case was to show Cheema had deceived Choongh into thinking there was no relationship between him and Singh and to implicate Singh's brother-in-law Varinder in the killing of Cheema.

Sir Desmond de Silva QC led the defence. Cross examining Gurjeet Choongh, he asked her to read several romantic text messages sent by Cheema to Singh after the engagement to Choongh. These he put to the witness showed, 'that it looks as though he was cheating on you behind your back' to which Choongh agreed, admitting that she was deeply hurt. It also emerged that Cheema was with Singh over the Christmas holidays only week before he was killed. The barrister put it to Choongh that 'Cheema had really told you a number of lies, the principal one of which was that you would be the only one in his life after the engagement'. Sir Desmond then had Choongh agree that Cheema's behaviour could be seen as a 'scandal' by some Sikh families and that Cheema's brother-in-law Varinder had spoken to her hours before Cheema's death. 'Was he angry and swearing a lot?' asked the barrister. 'Did he use the words, 'I am going to cover my hands with Lucky's blood and only then my aggression and my anger will calm down'. Choongh replied affirmatively. Sir Desmond stated, 'At 1 p.m. on January 27 Varinder was making, quite clearly, a threat to kill'.

The prosecution was led by Edward Brown QC who told the court that Singh poisoned the couple owing to 'jealousy, anger and revenge'. The court heard that two lodgers saw Singh entering Cheema's house before putting something in the refrigerated curry on the day of the killing. Also, a plastic bag containing powder had been found in Singh's coat which she claimed was medication for a neck rash. It was in fact aconite, the poison found in the curry.

On 10 February, 2010 Singh was convicted of Cheema's murder and of grievous bodily harm against his fiancé. The Crown pressed for a life sentence with a minimum of 30 years given that there were two victims, and the level of premeditation was high. Lakhvir Singh was jailed for at least 23 years. Judge Paul Worsley told the Singh that she would be approaching 70 before she could be considered for parole. He told her 'You were not just a spurned lover, you did not simply explode with anger at the rejection. You set about a cold and calculating revenge'.

Points of Special Interest

The case is notable for the degree of planning, involving Singh travelling to India to procure aconite. Physical evidence of the poison found in Singh's possession matching that in the curry and a witness to Singh removing the dish from the refrigerator were important. Motive was also evident as a combination of anger, jealousy and a desire for revenge. Time constraints within which Singh had to act are clear in that she intended to remove Cheema before he could marry his fiancé.

The defence case was an example of admitting that poison had been administered and that the intention was to kill, but that it was not the defendant that tampered with the food, but the deceased's brother-in-law whom it was said had threatened to kill the victim to preserve family honour.

Kristin Rossum, US

The Case

While at high school in California, Kristin Rossum used methamphetamine and other illegal drugs. Later moving to San Diego, she met Greg de Villier and appeared to overcome addictive use of methamphetamine. She graduated with honours with a degree in chemistry from San Diego State University in 1998. A year later she began work at San Diego County Medical Examiner's Office as a toxicologist. Marrying de Villiers in 1999, she began an affair with her manager Australian Michael Robertson in 2000.

Police reports indicate that on the morning of 6 November, the day de Villiers died, Rossum telephoned his office to say he would not be coming in that day and that he was asleep. She then went to work herself. Returning around lunchtime she found her husband awake but groggy and they shared soup. She then left again. Terry Huang his boss telephoned the de Villiers La Jolla home at 7 p.m. that day and Rossum told him that her husband was sleeping. An hour later, she telephoned 911 reporting that de Villiers was not breathing. When paramedics arrived, they found de Villiers unresponsive lying on the couple's bed surrounded by rose petals in a scene reminiscent of the movie 'American Beauty'. On arrival at hospital de Villiers was pronounced dead, his wife claiming that he had committed suicide.

It emerged that de Villiers had discovered about his wife's affair with Robertson and her relapse into drug use and had threatened to reveal both facts to the Medical Examiner's Office if Rossum did not leave her job. It appeared that Robertson learned of this threat prior to de Villier's being killed. Jerome de Villiers, Greg's brother was convinced that Greg was not suicidal. A month after de Villier's death, Rossum was fired for hiding her drug addiction, and Robertson dismissed for concealing Rossum's habit, and their affair. Concerned about possible conflict of interest in an employee carrying out an autopsy on an employee's husband, the San Diego County Medical Examiner Brian Blackburn arranged for de Villiers' autopsy to be carried out by an 'outside' laboratory in Los Angeles. Tests indicated seven times the lethal dose of fentanyl in de Villier's system. Samples were limited as immediately de Villiers was dead Rossum had donated his eyes and parts of his skin for transplant. These tend to be the most water retaining and therefore forensically useful body parts. But there was enough to determine cause of death as fentanyl.

Rossum told police that Greg had been depressed. She had suggested that they have trial separation. On the day before he died, she had telephone his employer to say that he would not be coming in. In June 2001, Rossum was arrested, charged with murder and released on bail.

At her trial, defence attorney Alex Loebig claimed that de Villiers had committed suicide by drinking fentanyl from a glass at his bedside that was never tested by police. There was no suicide note because de Villiers may have wanted revenge on his wife for her affair. The prosecution case put by Dan Goldstein was that Kristin had murdered her husband to prevent him revealing her affair and her drug thefts. The drinking theory did not explain that on Greg's body along with expected needle marks from the paramedics' treatment, there was an unaccounted for puncture where Kristin may have injected her husband with fentanyl. The rose petals may have been placed around the body by Kristin trying to create a melodramatic movie like scene. In marathon aspects to the trial, Rossum was on the witness stand for a total of over 8 h, prosecution closing arguments took over 7 h, and jury deliberated for 8 h.

Found guilty in November 2002, Rossum was subsequently sentenced to life imprisonment without the possibility of parole. Robertson returned to Australia after his employment was terminated. He was named in Rossum's trial as a co-conspirator.

Points of Special Interest

As in many poison trials much of the evidence was circumstantial but was considered by the jury sufficient to convict. There are relatively many medic-patient poisonings, because of a combination of access to potentially poisonous drugs, knowledge of their action and access to patients for treatment. In this case, the murderer had access to poisons and detailed knowledge of their action. Access to the victim was not through a physician–patient relationship but through being a spouse. Also it appears that Rossum would have known that her laboratory and autopsy services would not routinely test for fentanyl and so believed that it would go undetected.

The important spotting of the 'extra' needle mark on de Villier's body is reminiscent of the needle puncture noticed on the body of Elizabeth Barlow injected with insulin by her husband Kenneth Barlow [63] before he drowned her in her bath.

The issue of the autopsy being compromised was addressed by using an outside source, making the evidence impartial. As far as motive was concerned, the probability of Rossum seeking self-protection outweighed the possibility of de Villier's suicide.

Jessica Wongso. Australia and Indonesia

The Case

Jessica Wongso and Wayan Salihin an Australian resident attended design college together in Sydney Australia. Both were graphic designers. Jessica, her parents and two siblings emigrated from Indonesia to Australia in 2008 and are all permanent residents of Australia living in Sydney. In 2016, Jessica was an administrator in the New South Wales ambulance service from 2014 until she resigned in November 2015. It appears that in late 2015, Jessica and her parents returned to Indonesia for a vacation and were due to return to Australia in late January 2016.

On 6 January 2016, Jessica Wongso and Wayan Salihin met along with another friend for an afternoon coffee date at the Olivier café in the Grand Indonesia shopping mall, Jakarta, Indonesia. Wayan Salihin, after one sip of her iced Vietnamese coffee, collapsed suddenly, dying hours later in hospital. Jessica Wongso was arrested in late January, three weeks after the café meeting.

Closed-circuit television footage from inside the restaurant on Jan. 6 showed Jessica Wongso arriving about an hour before Wayan Salihin and the third woman. After sitting in a booth, she ordered drinks for the three of them. Footage showed Ms. Wongso putting her three shopping bags on the table, blocking her and the drinks from the camera's view. After making a series of unknown movements, she placed the bags on the seat. In June 2016, in court in Indonesia, prosecutors argued that the defendant laced Ms. Salihin's iced coffee with cyanide from behind her makeshift screen. The motive it was alleged was Wongso's jealousy of Salihin's relationship with her new husband. Also, Salihin had apparently disapproved of a relationship between Wongso and an Australian Patrick O'Connor which has recently ended. It was unclear how the cyanide was obtained but prosecution lawyers suggested that it was available on the black market.

The court ruled that Jessica Wongso killed her friend by spiking her drink. Judging that the poisoning was 'sadistic' the court sentenced Wongso to 20 years in prison.

Points of Special Interest

This is a rare female-on-female poisoning. It is also unusual in that a public place was chosen for what is usually a surreptitious crime. Indeed, secrecy was involved in the concealing from the CCTV camera the movements that Wongso made with the coffee on the café table. But the real camouflage it appears was that Wongso thought that there was safety in committing the crime in plain sight.

Conclusion

Cases from the US, UK and Indonesia were examined and points of particular relevance were identified.

Suggested Activity

Begin to familiarise yourself with the glossary. Look at the cases mentioned in the present chapter and see how they are outlined: Harold Shipman [81], Kristin Rossum [82], Lynn Turner [88], Lakhvir Singh [93], Paul Marshall Curry [95], Roger and David Cooper [99] and Jessica Wongso [100].

Reference

The Shipman Inquiry First Report. (2002, July) *Volume 1—Death Disguised; Volume 2—Decisions Todmorden; Volumes 3–6—Decisions Hyde.*

Chapter 3
Criminal Poisoning in Theory

Theories and Explanations

There is no shortage of interest in homicide in news outlets or in movies for as Hough and McCorkle (2017) reminds us, 'murder continues to fascinate' (Ibid. p. 2). But what of theory? In an apocryphal tale, a student is discussing a research proposition with his professor. Presenting a clear picture of the practicalities of the research, the student grows increasingly exasperated that his mentor keeps asking more and more questions. Eventually the professor explains. 'I see perfectly well what you want to do in practice. What you haven't explained yet, is how you intend to do it in theory'. If I understand the point of this story correctly, it is that although the nuts and bolts of an undertaking are important and often quickly apparent, the theoretical aspects are equally relevant but may not always be so clear. So the question arises, 'Is there a theory or a set of theories that can clarify and begin to explain the phenomenon of homicidal poisoning?'

In addressing this question we need to look at biological, psychological, and sociological levels of explanations of crime. It will be clear that none of them in isolation offers a comprehensive explanation but that interaction is likely to take place between factors at these different levels. Examining each approach however allows us to see how much light it throws on homicide and on homicidal poisoning.

Biological Theories of Crime

Heredity and Genetics

Twin studies and adoption research have explored possible inherited components to crime. Twin studies compare levels of criminality between genetically identical (monozygotic of MZ) twins, and non-identical (dizygotic or DZ) twins who are no

M. Farrell, *Criminology of Homicidal Poisoning*,
DOI 10.1007/978-3-319-59117-9_3

more similar in their genetic make-up than ordinary siblings. It is reasoned that if criminality levels are more similar for MZ twins than for DZ twins (that is if there is a greater rate of 'concordance' between MZ than DZ twins for criminal behaviour), this constitutes evidence of genetic inheritance and crime. Summaries of this research are available in various textbooks (e.g. Williams 2001). Researchers' interpretations of their findings range from concluding that there is no evidence of inherited criminality, to claims that there are clear indications of inheritance. Others take a more nuanced position somewhere in between. In effect, the current state of knowledge shows a mixed picture.

Adoption studies seek to apportion the relative influences of inheritance and environment (including upbringing) by comparing the criminality of adopted individuals with that of their biological and their adoptive parents. Often cited is the series of longitudinal Danish Adoption Studies (Mednick et al. 1987). These compared the criminal records of adopted children with those of their biological and their adoptive parents. Some 13% of children had a criminal record when neither their biological nor their adoptive father had a record. Where the adoptive father had been convicted of crime, the percentage rose to 14.7%. In instances where the biological father had committed a crime it was 20%. A figure of 24.5% was found when both natural and adoptive fathers were offenders. Cautiously, the researchers claim that the findings indicate that inherited traits may lead to certain individuals in particular environments being more prone to criminality than individuals in the same situation who do not have these inherited traits. Just as with twin studies the interpretations of such adoption studies are debated.

As Brookman (2005) indicates, most reviews of twin and adoption studies accept that although genetics may have a contributory role in criminality, it is 'in conjunction with environmental and social influences' (Ibid. p. 51).

Brain Glucose Metabolism

It is suggested that abnormal brain processes can predispose certain individuals to violent crime. Some 22 murderers and attempted murderers were matched with control subjects. The 'murderer' sample were all pleading insanity as their defence, making then a very distinctive group. Positron emission tomography scanning indicated that murderers had much reduced glucose metabolism in the pre-frontal cortex than controls (Raine et al. 1994). Similar results were later found with an expanded group of murderers and controls.

Neurotransmitters

Neurotransmitters, for example serotonin, dopamine, and norepinephrine, are chemicals facilitating the passage of electrical nerve impulses. Serotonin can inhibit responses to emotional stimuli thereby reducing aggressiveness. Dopamine and norepinephrine on the other hand have an excitatory effect counteracting serotonin's inhibitory influence. Imbalances in these neurotransmitters has been linked to aggression leading to the suggestion that individuals with lower than typical levels of serotonin may be prone to violent or impulsive behaviour (Fishbein 1996).

Brain Anomalies—The Amygdala

Examining certain physiological processes that could predispose some criminals to violent behaviour, Raine, Buchsbaum and LaCasse (1997) looked at murderers pleading not guilty by reason of insanity. They suggest that among the many predispositions to violence for such individuals is reduced activity in prefrontal, parietal and callosal brain regions. Also implicated were asymmetries in the activity of the thalamus, amygdala, and medial temporal lobe. Reduced activity in the prefrontal areas may be associated with impulsiveness, poor self-control, immaturity, altered emotionality, and being unable to modify behaviour. With all of these anomalies, normal limitations on behaviour may be reduced, increasing the likelihood of aggressive acts. It appears that deficits in several of these processes is necessary in order to cumulatively increase the likelihood of violence.

Psychological Theories of Crime

Criminological psychology has been defined as, 'the application of psychological theory and investigation to understanding (and attempting to change) criminal behaviour' (Hollin 2012, p. 81). But what do such psychological theories suggest?

Developments in a Freudian Tradition

Sigmund Freud (1856–1939), identifying tensions between the prohibitions of 'civilisation' and instinctual desires, suggests that, among the 'instinctual wishes' is a 'lust for killing' (Freud [1927]/2001, p. 10). Discussing prohibitions that forbid these wishes he adds, 'The instinctual wishes that suffer under them [the prohibitions] are born afresh with every child' (Ibid.). Following Freud's psychoanalytic framework, Austrian psychoanalyst August Aichhorn (1878–1949) presented his ideas in *Wayward Youth* (Aichhorn [1925]/1961) which had a forward by Freud himself. Aichhorn regarded juvenile crime as the result of 'latent delinquency', a sort of psychological disposition. Drawing on Freud's proposed 'pleasure principle' (Freud [1920]/2001, pp. 7–66), in which behaviour is based around pleasure-seeking, Aichhorn suggested that this latent delinquency became expressed as overt behaviour owing to failures in emotional development and socialisation.

British psychiatrist and psychoanalyst John Bowlby (1907–1990) valorised the bond between mother and child, which he termed 'attachment'. His theory of attachment relates to the biological survival of the species and functions to secure the infant's safety in a loving environment (Bowlby 1965, 1969, 1973, 1980). Five instinctive responses lead to greater 'proximity' to the mother and mediate attachment: sucking, smiling, clinging, crying, and following. The child's attachment to the mother does not derive from her providing for the child's needs, but is instinctual and primary. Bowlby's research into early experience of loss and separation indicated that they lead to mourning, reflecting the primacy of the child's bond with the mother. Emotional security, built up through experiences in early childhood, relates to the child's confidence in the availability of attachment figures. Different forms of anxiety mirror basic anxiety about the separation from the object of attachment. Such is the power of separation from the mother or rejection by her that it can lead to childhood problems and difficulties in later development, including delinquency (Please see www.thebowlbycentre.org.uk).

Differential Association Theory and Differential Reinforcement Theory

In developing differential association theory, American criminologist Edwin Sutherland (1853–1950) took account of social factors that define crime and the environment in which it most often takes place. Sutherland (1947) argued that, being set in a social context, criminal behaviour is essentially learned. Behaviour is learned in close social groups and is acquired by contacts with them. Where these groups are delinquent, it becomes more likely that the learning will involve acquiring skills associated with crime and forming attitudes necessary to sustain criminal behaviour.

Following on from Sutherland's references to learned behaviour, Jeffrey (1965) developed differential reinforcement theory. This drew on the operant conditioning work of the American behavioural psychologist B.F. Skinner (1904–1990) concerning the effects of reward, punishment and the avoidance of unpleasant circumstances on the frequency of the occurrence of behaviour (Skinner 1938). In differential reinforcement theory, criminal behaviour was seen as operant behaviour, being determined by the consequences that it created. For example, should a property crime be successful, the perpetrator is rewarded and this is likely to 'positively reinforce' the criminal behaviour so that it will occur more often. If someone suffers unpleasant circumstances such as poverty, then the successful acquisition of property through crime allows them to avoid straightened circumstances in a scenario of 'negative reinforcement'. This too increases the likelihood of the criminal behaviour being repeated. Risks of being caught and the consequences of a fine, imprisonment or other punishment act to reduce the likelihood that crime will be repeated. As well as such physical or material consequences, the theory accepts that social and personal consequences also act as encouragements or deterrents. Although this is a theory of crime in the broad sense, it might apply to some extent to crimes of violence where violent behaviour goes unpunished or is even rewarded from the perpetrator's viewpoint.

Eysenck's Theory of Crime

In a personality theory of crime, psychologist Hans Eysenck (1916–1997) took account of the interaction of biological, individual and social influences (Eysenck 1977). The theory holds that genetic inheritance leads to individual physiological differences in the cortical nervous system and autonomic nervous system. These in turn influence an individual's ability to learn from stimuli in the environment. Three personality dimensions are involved: extroversion-introversion, neuroticism-stability, and high psychoticism-low psychoticism. Each forms a continuum with most people being somewhere in the middle of each dimension.

An extrovert is cortically under-aroused, so seeks stimulation to gain optimum arousal. This is associated with taking risks, thrill seeking, and impulsiveness. An introvert is cortically under-aroused and therefore avoids stimulation to keep arousal at an acceptable level. Accordingly, the introvert is quiet and reserved and avoids risk and high levels of stimulation. Also extraverts, 'condition' less effectively than introverts.

An individual with high neuroticism has a highly labile autonomic nervous system so experiences strong reactions to unpleasant or painful stimuli. This translates to irritability, and anxious behaviour. Someone with low neuroticism has a stable autonomic nervous system and tends to be calm and unruffled.

High neuroticism is associated with poor conditioning because of the interfering effects of anxiety. Low neuroticism is linked to good conditionability. Those having a low N-low E profile will condition best while individuals with high N—high E will condition poorest. Individuals with high N-low E or high E-low N will be somewhere in between. These differing levels of conditionability lead to different levels of socialisation. High levels of psychoticism are associated with lack of fellow feeling, preference for solitude, aggressiveness, and tough-mindedness. Its possible physiological bases are unclear. A personality inventory was developed to assess the levels of the three dimensions. Socialisation is seen as a process which leads to acceptable behaviour and is related to successful conditioning. Where socialisation is less successful, deviant and criminal behaviour is expected to be more likely. Consequently in criminal populations, one would expect individuals to have high E and high N and (as P is associated with aggressiveness) high P also.

Empirical testing of Eysenck's theory indicated that groups of offenders tended as predicted to score highly on N and P, although scores for E were equivocal. Eysenck and Eysenck (1971) later suggested that offenders may have high levels of 'impulsiveness' and low levels of 'sociability' which could be masked in the overall E levels. Eysenck and McGurk (1980) found support for this hypothesis in that a sample of offenders scored higher than a non-offender group in impulsiveness but not in sociability. McGurk and McDougal (1981) found that the combinations of traits predicted by the theory to relate to criminal behaviour (high E and high N; and high P, high N, high E) typified a delinquent sample, while also as expected the highly socialised combination of low E and low N was found only in a non-offender sample.

Hollin (2012, p. 92) recognises the empirical evidence supporting Eysenck's theory but points out that the link between conditioning and socialisation is not always convincingly established. Eysenck's theory can be seen as a positivist and largely determinist theory (Farrell 1989e) taking insufficient account of the dynamic interaction between individual and society (Taylor et al. 1973). Also, it is unclear what effect overall levels of psychoticism are expected where criminals include a sub group of social inadequate rather than explicitly aggressive individuals (Farrell 1984, 1988a).

Cognitive Theories of Crime

Cognitive theories are concerned with the process of thinking and its influence on attitudes, beliefs and behaviour. Among such theories relating to crime are ones concerned with personal control and perceptions of control. Rotter (1966) (www.soc.iastate.edu/sapp/soc512Rotter.pdf) developed research on 'locus of control'. This concerned the extent to which an individual considered their behaviour was internal or external in its locus that is the degree to which it is under personal control. A person who was high on internal control believed that what happened to them was their responsibility. Those high on external control considered that what happened was down to luck or the influence of others. Several studies (e.g. Hollin and Wheeler 1982) have found that offenders tend towards an external locus of control, attributing their behaviour to outside influences. In the specific instance of homicide however, it appears that professional killers exert strong self-control supported by planning where they can to avoid prolonged contact with the victim (Collins 2009, p. 432).

Another relevant cognitive theory is the moral reasoning theory developed by Kohlberg (1978). He proposes that moral reasoning develops sequentially with maturity. Three levels are identified each with two stages.

- Level 1 is that of pre-morality with stages characterised by punishment and obedience; and by a hedonistic concern with one's own needs.
- Level 2 is typified by conventional conformity with a stage of interpersonal concordance (associated with social approval) and 'law and order' involving a commitment to law and order for its own sake.
- Level 3 has to do with autonomous principles. Its two stages involve social contract, and universal ethical principles.

As will be noticed, the stages move from the concrete to the more abstract as the individual matures. For Kohlberg, offending is associated with delays in the development of moral reasoning so that when the opportunity to offend arises, an individual lacks reasoning power to resist the temptation. Indeed, moral reasoning has been associated with criminal conduct (Palmer 2003).

Within the context of a model of social information processing (Crick and Dodge 1994), it is found that aggressive individuals tend to look for and perceive fewer social cues than non-violent individuals (Dodge and Newman 1981). Such aggressive people also interpret inter-personal cues as hostile (Slaby and Guerra 1988).

Sociological Theories of Crime

Functionalism

Among examples of sociological theories related to crime is functionalism, which concerns itself with social systems. Participants in social action are not necessarily aware of the role that their conduct plays. Deviance is seen not as a force that disrupts social order but one which works in ways to maintain it. Applied to crime, it was suggested for example that racketeering on the New York docks offered alternative routes to success and contributed to social stability (Bell 1960).

Anomie

'Anomie' (normlessness) influenced by the work of French sociologist Emile Durkheim (1858–1917) (Durkheim [1893]/1964 and [1897]/1952) has been cited to suggest that crime thrives when social disorganisation is so pronounced that society approaches a state of collapse. Anomie could be experienced as so disillusioning and debilitating that it could lead people to 'commit suicide and homicide' (Lukes 1967, p. 139). Of wider application is another path of these theories that crime develops owing to flawed social regulation which provides few restraints and little moral direction.

Merton (1938) argued that crime arises owing to a tension between society's cultural goals and structural social limitations. US citizens had been encouraged to work for financial success, yet lower class individuals were often prevented from reaching such goals through educational or employment routes. Some individuals would continue to conform to ideals of monetary success despite not performing well. Others would respond to the strain and frustration through deviant reactions. One of these, 'innovation' tended to be associated with crime: the individual remains committed to gaining wealth but adopts deviant means such as robbery to do so (Ibid.). In its most florid forms anomie can involve the collapse of a social order and extreme violence as for example with the militant Islamist group Boko Haram in Nigeria (Rock 2012, and personal communication, 2017).

The approach contributed to the development of 'strain theory' (Farrell 1991a). Subsequently, adaptations of strain theory have maintained that crime could be precipitated through tensions other than frustrated goals of wealth but also of status and self-reliance (e.g. Agnew 2001). As Brookman (2005) observes, this inclusion of strain relating to striving for status as well as monetary goals gives the theory a wider applicability to homicide (Ibid. pp. 103–104).

Control Theory

In control theory, an implication is that many people would commit crimes if there were not inducements to comply with social rules. Hirschi (1969) suggested four inducements to rule compliance: attachment, commitment, involvement and belief. Attachment for example, was concerned with the extent to which an individual was responsive to the opinions of others.

Among the many variations and applications of control theory is that described in *Shared Beginnings Divergent Lives* (Laub and Sampson 2003). This concerns the life course of men followed over many years, looking at how delinquency was resisted or accepted. It examined, among other things, the way that social bonds such as friends, family, military service and employment act as informal controls, and filter influences existing in the wider social structure. Among complications for such a view is when crimes including illegal homicide and rape are committed by military personnel (see for example Beevor 2002).

Rational Choice Theory

Rational choice theory, echoing utilitarian philosophy, suggests that people make rational choices about committing crime based on opportunity and risks in a similar way that they make other life choices. Relatedly the rate of crime is considered to be responsive to factors which influence such decisions. For example Clarke (1992) delineates groups of factors that can influence crime. These configurations made it harder to commit the crime, or made it riskier to commit the crime, or reduced the rewards of crime (Ibid. p. 13). In the first group of factors for example is 'controlling facilitators' such as gun control which would be expected to cut down firearm crime. As well as a sociological level, concerning opportunities for crime according to variables in the environment, this theory also implies a particular psychological view of individuals as being able to reason and to calculate risks.

Routine Activities Theory

In posing the question of how criminal activity might be limited or prevented by the regular activities of daily life, routine activities theory (Felson 1994) suggests that crime is motivated, discouraged, and otherwise shaped by the warp and weft of everyday life. Conversant with this theory, it might be expected that increases in the availability of valuable, portable goods such as laptop computers and smart phones will increase the incidence of stealing.

Chicago School

The sociology department of the University of Chicago developed, from the 1920s, approaches involving social ecology and urban mapping that were highly influential to later criminology (e.g. Park 1925). As cities grew, it was suggested, space, people and function would be differentiated so that different groupings would form in different areas or 'zones'. This would happen in an organic sort of way, largely spontaneously. In the city of Chicago itself, various zones were identified including a 'zone of transition' having distinctive characteristics such as weak social control and fast physical change. Mapping social problems in the area showed that it had higher proportions than other areas of problems such as poverty, poor educational levels, and juvenile delinquency.

A further development of this school was the study of the customs and practices of residents of the natural areas of the city. A degree of social and moral dislocation was found in the zone of transition and between that zone and the rest of society. But researchers also found evidence of cohesiveness and a continuity of culture and behaviour. This continued across generations and immigrant groups within the same area over time. Delinquency was a continuing aspect of life and 'traditions of delinquency were preserved and transmitted' for example through delinquent gangs (Shaw 1971).

Subsequently, as the social mapping of offenders was recognised as important, the similar mapping of offences was explored. One finding was of crime 'hot spots' in Minneapolis where for example 3% of all places produced 50% of calls to the police (Sherman et al. 1989, p. 27). Other developments in criminology relating to the impact of space, and of surveillance are summarised by Rock (2012, pp. 56–59).

Radical Criminology and Left Realism

Radical criminology, sometimes known as 'new criminology' or 'critical criminology' was concerned with issues of politics, control, and power and with inequalities in society (Farrell 1990d). In some versions it was rooted in Marxism

(Taylor et al. 1973). After a brief period of influence in the 1960s and 1970s, radical criminology led to left realism (Young 1997). This moved away from emphasising that crime was bound up with ideology, and accepted the real impact of crime on people especially the poor in society.

Labelling Theory

In considering labelling theory, it is first necessary to touch on two contributions to it: phenomenology and symbolic interactionism. Phenomenology is philosophical perspective with different emphases. For example the transcendental phenomenology of Husserl ([1913a]/1980, [1913b]/1982, [1913c]/1989) maintains that although the independent existence of things can be questioned, what cannot be doubted is how things appear to us immediately in consciousness. Therefore knowledge should be based on these phenomenal experiences (Please also see Farrell 2012, pp. 49–53). Symbolic interactionism, a sociological perspective of self and society, takes many forms. Essentially, people are regarded as living their lives in a symbolic environment. Symbols are seen as social objects that are derived from culture, and their meaning is shared and developed in interaction with others. Language allows symbols to act as the means by which reality is constructed, largely as a social product. The sense of self, society and culture emerge from symbolic interactions. Indeed they depend on symbolic interaction for their existence. Physical environment is interpreted through symbolic systems in the way it is made relevant to human behaviour (Ibid. pp. 145–148).

These ideas are applied to deviant acts and identities, leading to an emphasis on the ways in which these are constructed, interpreted, evaluated, and controlled over time. In the process of developing a 'career' of deviance, the importance of language became a key aspect of labelling theory. Labelling that takes place in the criminal justice system was considered to have particular power and authority. An individual commits an initial delinquent act (the so called 'primary deviance'). They experience the reactions of others identifying them as deviant. The individual may respond in a deviant role for examples as a means of defence or attack. If so the deviance becomes, 'secondary', incorporating the knowledge, stereotypes, and experience of others in shaping identity and future behaviour. (e.g. Becker 1963).

Sub Culture

A social group which persists over time, shares common goals and perhaps common problems, may form, take over or modify a 'subculture' (Rock 2012, p. 68, paraphrased) Criminology is especially interested in subcultures which, 'condone, promote, and otherwise make possible the commission of delinquent acts' (Ibid.). An example of work on subculture is the study of delinquent boys by Cohen

(1957). Many of the orientations in criminology have looked at sub cultures and sought to explain them in terms of their theories. Anomie theory, the Chicago School, control theory, symbolic interaction, and radical criminology have all done so. For example, in a symbolic interactionist view, subcultures were examined in terms of the negotiation and group agreement of meaning. (For a classic exposition concerning subculture see Ferracuti and Wolfgang ([1967]/2010).

Feminism

Links between feminism and criminology have been recognised for some time (e.g. Gelsthorpe and Morris 1988). Indeed, the influence of feminism on criminology has been seen in the growing volume of work on women as offenders and victims, the role of women in the criminal justice system, and an interest in 'masculinity' and why much crime appears to be the preserve of males. Snider (1998) suggests that violence towards women is sustained through ideology and social structure relating to capitalism and patriarchy which in turn influences dominant male identity. She proposes that, '…it must be possible to find ways of being manly that are not misogynous and do not require the repression of every human emotion except anger' (Ibid. p. 24). Others have paid greater attention to the differences within conceptions of masculinity and femininity (Walklate 2001).

Among recent books of interest are *Women, Murder and Femininity* (Seal 2010) focusing on murders in mid nineteenth century England and Wales. *Murder, Gender and the Media* (Monkton-Smith 2012) includes chapters concerning intimate partner abuse and intimate partner femicide. Regarding poisoning, *Nineteenth Century Female Poisoners* (Nagy 2015) looks at three cases in detail.

Theories of Crime in Relation to Poisoning Homicide

Biological Theories of Crime in Relation to Poisoning Homicide

The possibility of there being a hereditary component to property crime and similar deviance seems far-fetched because the crime is carried out in such an obviously contrived social context that it seems antipathetic to notions of hereditary influence. More plausible is the idea that explosive physical violence might have a hereditary element. Yet when one comes to consider poison homicide, the possible influence of inheritance seems implausible because the violence involved is not of the explosive physical contact type. More broadly, most reviews of twin and adoption studies accept that although genetics may have a contributory role in criminality, it is 'in conjunction with environmental and social influences' (Brookman 2005, p. 51).

The possible relevance to homicidal poisoning of reduced glucose metabolism in the pre-frontal cortex of murderers is limited by the fact that it was found a small group of murderers who had pleased an insanity defence, none of whom it seems were charged with poison murder (Raine et al. 1994).

Imbalances in the neurotransmitters serotonin, dopamine, and norepinephrine has been linked to aggressive behaviour, while individuals with lower than usual levels of serotonin may be prone to violent or impulsive behaviour (Fishbein 1996). However with poison murder the behaviour tends not to be impulsive but secretive and calculating, making it difficult to see any application of these findings. Similar reservations arise when considering brain anomalies and psychophysiological processes that could predispose some criminals to violent behaviour (e.g. Raine et al. 1997).

Biological influences may account for some of the influences on violence. But any such effects are not simple and related to individual brain processes and deficits. They are complex and likely to involve several processes cumulatively in interaction with other influences (such as psychological and social ones). Also biological explanations relating to physical changes in violent individuals cannot explain changes in the rates of violence over centuries and decades (e.g. Spierenburg 2008; Eisner 2014).

Psychological Theories of Crime in Relation to Poisoning Homicide

Aichhorn ([1925]/1961) regarded juvenile crime as the result of 'latent delinquency', suggesting that this became expressed as overt behaviour owing to failures in emotional development and socialisation. In Bowlby's theory of 'attachment' (Bowlby 1965, 1969, 1973, 1980) separation from the mother or rejection by her can lead to childhood problems and difficulties in later development, including delinquency. While such ideas and related research has informed provision for very disturbed children and adolescents (Dockar-Drysdale 1968, 1973, 1990) its relevance to any specific crime of homicidal poisoning is unclear.

For Sutherland (1947) criminal behaviour in its social context is learned in close social groups and is acquired by contacts with such groups which (when these are delinquent) involves learning skills associated with crime and the attitudes supporting criminal behaviour (see also, Farrell 1988b). Relatedly, in differential reinforcement theory (Jeffrey 1965) criminal behaviour and its frequency is seen as determined by the consequences it creates whether positive or negative. This could have relevance to poison murder where poison is administered over a period of several days or weeks and the perpetrator goes undetected so that they are reinforced in their actions. With serial poisoners too, such positive and negative consequences could increase the chances of the poisoner repeating the offense with other victims. Very occasionally where there are cases of two or more people acting together to poison (team poisoning) there may be social and personal encouragement to poison again, as well as material reasons. Care is needed especially regarding team poisoning in suggesting broad theories or explanations because its extreme rarity may mean that there are idiosyncratic causes that do not lend themselves to broad explanations.

Eysenck's (1977) personality theory of crime takes account of the interaction of biological, individual and social influences. In line with predictions, empirical testing of Eysenck's theory indicated that groups of offenders tended to score highly on N and P, although scores for E were equivocal. Eysenck and Eysenck (1971) later suggested that offenders may have high 'impulsiveness' and low 'sociability' which could be masked in the overall E levels which appears to have been confirmed (Eysenck and McGurk 1980). Also combinations of traits predicted by the theory to be related to criminal behaviour (high E and high N; and high P, high N, high E) were found only in a delinquent sample (McGurk and McDougal 1981). So what might be the personality profile of poisoners? Poisoners might have high levels of psychoticism indicating lack of fellow feeling. But the high N (which with high E that seems to relate to conditionability and crime) would not be expected. This is because the crime of poisoning is typically not one of impulsivity, but of careful calculation. While such observations might give an indication of expected personality profiles in terms of Eysenck's theory, they would not be conversant with the mechanics of the theory in its efforts to explain crime through conditioning.

Following Rotter (1966) studies (e.g. Hollin and Wheeler 1982) have found that offenders tend towards an external locus of control, explaining their behaviour as being predominantly owing to outside influences. To the extent that poisoners tend to calculate and plan ahead, they are less likely to see their actions as being the responsibility of others. Indeed it is the very act of control that appears to influence some sadistic poisonings and chronic poisoning in which the perpetrator can choose to prolong a victim's suffering.

For Kohlberg (1978) offending is associated with delays in the development of moral reasoning so that when the opportunity to offend arises, an individual lacks a sufficient level of reasoning to resist the temptation. Moral reasoning has also been associated with criminal conduct (Palmer 2003). Although a criminal poisoner has to plan and reason in order to carry out their crime, this does not necessarily imply a good level of *moral* reasoning, indeed being able to watch over extended periods the suffering of others whom one is poisoning suggests a lack of moral reasoning and feeling.

It appears that aggressive individuals tend to look for and perceive fewer social cues than non-violent individuals (Dodge and Newman 1981) and interpret inter-personal cues in a hostile way (Slaby and Guerra 1988). However this seems to apply to confrontational violence rather than to the planning and calculated actions of poisoning.

Sociological Theories of Crime in Relation to Poisoning Homicide

Many theories of crime in general focused on relatively frequent offences against property are not always applicable to homicide. Routine activities theory (Felson 1994) is an example. Functionalism has echoes in today's criminology but its notion that crime has a function in making society cohesive goes against strong intuitive views (and empirical evidence).

Never the less some theories appear to have potential if limited relevance as with the idea that in extreme cases of social disintegration, anomie can be experienced as so disillusioning and debilitating that it can precipitate suicide and murder (Lukes 1967, p. 139). Rational choice theory, can concern factors which influence such decisions to commit or not to commit criminal activities such as 'controlling facilitators' (Clarke 1992, p. 13). Just as, in this theory, gun control is expected to reduce gun crime, so controls on the sale and use of poisons would be expected to reduce poison homicide. In fact, data indicates such a reduction in England following the implementation of the *Arsenic Act 1851* and subsequent related Acts which cut down poison-related crime particularly concerning arsenic (Watson 2004, p. 43).

The social ecology and urban mapping of the Chicago School (e.g. Park 1925) may have relevance to the study of crimes committed regularly, including homicides in particular geographical areas. Never the less, they may have less relevance for the comparatively rare crime of poison murder. Control theory seems applicable to so called 'life course' studies and careers of delinquency (or its rejection) in the light of social bonds and other influences over a considerable period (Laub and Sampson 2003). Therefore it may have relevance to understanding chronic homicidal poisoning and may shed light on serial poison murder where habits of killing may develop over time.

Labelling theory (Becker 1963) seems to explain something of an individual's shifts in identity and behaviour over time as they become influenced by 'secondary deviance' in a career of delinquency. It may apply to serial poisoning where the offender sees and hears accounts of their crimes for example in the mass media. They may then, as time passes, shape their offending according the responses they elicit. This interpretation is different to how labelling theory is normally understood. The individual is not directly confronted by the views and reaction to themselves, but experience it secretly through channels such as the media and what they hear others saying about the crimes. Work on subculture (e.g. Cohen 1957) may have relevance in the rare circumstances when more than one perpetrator is involved in poison murder, when the meaning of the deviant behaviour may be mutually mitigated by the offenders. Feminism and a 'gendered' view of crime (e.g. Gelsthorpe and Morris 1988) may shed light on homicidal poisoning, for example in exploring issues around role expectations of women.

'Strain theory' suggests that crime arises owing to a tension between society's cultural goals and structural social limitations relating to financial aspirations

(Merton 1938) or more widely to strivings for status and self-reliance (Agnew 2001). Both these aspects may have application to homicide (Brookman 2005, pp. 103–104). With regard to poison killings too, such explanations may apply to some cases.

Promising Theories for Poisoning Homicide

Some 'Types' of Poisoning

Current biological theories appear to offer little to explain of homicidal poisoning. Some seek to explain violent or impulsive behaviour (Fishbein 1996) but this is not typical of poison homicides. Of the psychological and the sociological theories discussed, several may have relevance to poisoning homicide. In reviewing these, I want to distinguish some types of poisoning that will be discussed in more detail in later chapters, and also include a broader category of 'poisoning in general' as follows:

- 'Poisoning in general' (this does not necessarily exclude chronic, serial, or team poisoning but may apply to poisoning more generally)
- Serial poisoning (where several victims are poisoned one after the other over a period of time with a 'cooling off' period between killings)
- 'Team poisoning' where two or more perpetrators act together.

Poisoning in General

If offending is associated with delays in the development of moral reasoning, then when the opportunity to offend arises, an individual may lack the reasoning to resist the temptation of poisoning (Kohlberg 1978). Clearly, lack of moral reasoning does not preclude the ability to reason in general and plan ahead to perpetrate the poisoning.

Rational choice theory (Clarke 1992) may help explain factors which influence decisions to commit or desist from criminal activities for example 'controlling facilitators' such as controls on the sale and use of poisons. As a method of killing, the choice of poisoning is rational in the sense that with other methods, one can make the death appear accidental or suicidal. But with poisoning, as well as these possibilities, there is the possibility of making death appear to be owing to natural causes for example illness, disease or simply expected death from old age.

Aspects of feminism and a 'gendered' view of crime (e.g. Gelsthorpe and Morris 1988) may have relevance for homicidal poisoning for example in examining the gender of perpetrators and victims.

The 'strain theory' that crime arises from tension between society's cultural goals and structural social limitations relating to financial aspirations (Merton 1938) or to strivings for status and self-reliance (Agnew 2001) may apply to homicide (Brookman 2005, pp. 103–104) including some poison killings.

Serial Poisoning

Differential reinforcement theory (Jeffrey 1965), in which criminal behaviour and its frequency is determined by the positive or negative consequences it creates could have relevance to undetected serial poisoning so that the perpetrator is reinforced in their actions.

Control theory seems applicable to so called 'life course' studies and careers of delinquency (or its rejection) in the light of social bonds and other influences over a considerable period (Laub and Sampson 2003) and this may be relevant to understanding serial poisoning.

Labelling theory (Becker 1963) may apply in some degree to serial poisoning where the offender witnesses accounts of their crimes in the mass media and over time shape their offending according to the way that they are depicted. The individual is not directly confronted by the views and reaction to themselves, but experience it secretly through the media and what others around them unknowingly say about the crimes.

Team Poisoning

Work on subculture (e.g. Cohen 1957) may be relevant to poison murder when more than one person is involved in the homicide and the meaning of the deviant behaviour is mutually mitigated by the offenders.

Conclusion

In reviewing the theoretical frameworks for crime including violent crime and homicide, no comprehensive overall theory is evident (or perhaps even possible). There is no philosopher's stone of crime (Farrell 1989a). Neither is there a comprehensive theory for poison homicide. There are however areas where the outlines of an understanding of poison homicide can be discerned. These include contributions from psychological and sociological theorising and research and relate to poisoning in general serial poisoning, and team poisoning.

Perhaps the most promising theme running through the theoretical possibilities discussed in this chapter is that of the shaping of behaviour and understanding over time. For example rational choice theory (Clarke 1992) concerns factors which influence decisions to commit or desist from criminal activities. In line with this, poisoning is a rational choice because unlike other methods such as shooting or stabbing it can allow death to appear to be from natural causes.

With regard to differential reinforcement theory (Jeffrey 1965), serial poisoning and its frequency is determined by the positive or negative consequences it creates. Labelling theory (Becker 1963) may shape the offenders view of themselves and their subsequent behaviour especially with regard to serial poisoning. With team poisoning, the shaping of meaning and the behaviour itself is related to the mutual subcultural (Cohen 1957) mitigation of the crime.

When someone poisons, the distinctive aspect of the crime is the planning and calculation that is associated with it, implying a self-directed shaping of events. Consistent with this is that the poisoner would be influenced by factors that contribute to the shaping of behaviour and understanding. Also where there is serial poisoning the opportunity for shaping behaviour and understanding (and meaning) is even more sustained. With team poisoning, the shaping of meaning and behaviour is likely to be amplified because it is reciprocated in the perpetrating offenders.

Suggested Activity

From the glossary, find examples of each of: individual poisoning, serial poisoning and team poisoning.

Key Texts

Brookman (2005) *Understanding Homicide*. London and Los Angeles, Sage.

Dealing with the criminology of homicide, this book discusses regarding homicide contexts, explanations, forms (such as male or female perpetrators, and multiple homicide), investigation and prevention.

Hough and McCorkle (2017) *American Homicide*. Thousand Oaks, CA and London, Sage.

This well-structured and engagingly written book includes a chapter 'Why We Do It: Theories of Homicide'.

Maguire et al. (2012) (5th edition) *The Oxford Handbook of Criminology*. Oxford, Oxford University Press.

This book covers: criminological history and theory of crime; social constructions of crime and crime control; dimensions of crime (such as gender and ethnicity); forms of crime; and reactions to crime (including sentencing, prevention and policing).

References

Agnew, R. (2001). Strain theory. In E. McLaughlin, & J. Muncie (Eds.), *The sage dictionary of criminology*. London: Sage.

Aichhorn, A. ([1925]/1961). *Wayward youth: A psychoanalytical study of delinquent children illustrated by actual case histories*. Cleveland, Meridian Books (Translated from the German) Becker, H. (1963) *Outsiders*. New York: Free Press.

Becker, H. (1963). *Outsiders*. New York: Free Press.

Beevor, A. (2002). *Berlin: The downfall 1945*. New York and London: Viking Press/Penguin.

Bell, D. (1960). The Racket Ridden Longshoremen. In *The end of ideology: On the exhaustion of political ideas in the fifties*. New York: Collier.

Bowlby, J. (1965). *Child care and the growth of love* (2nd ed.). Harmondsworth: Penguin Books.

Bowlby, J. (1969). *Attachment and loss volume 1—Attachment*. London: Hogarth Press.

Bowlby, J. (1973). *Attachment and loss volume 2—Separation, anxiety and anger*. London: Hogarth Press.

Bowlby, J. (1980). *Attachment and loss volume 3—Loss, sadness and depression*. London: Hogarth Press.

Brookman, F. (2005). *Understanding homicide*. London and Los Angeles: Sage.

Clarke, R. V. (Ed.). (1992). *Situational crime prevention: Successful case studies*. New York: Harrow and Heston.

Cohen. A. (1957). *Delinquent boys*. Glencoe: Free Press.

Collins, R. (2009). *Violence: A micro-sociological theory*. Princeton, NJ: Princeton University Press.

Crick, N. R., & Dodge, K. A. (1994). A review and reformulation of social information-processing mechanisms in children's social adjustment. *Psychological Bulletin, 115*, 74–101.

Dockar-Drysdale, B. (1968). *Therapy in child care*. London: Longman.

Dockar-Drysdale, B. (1973). *Consultations in child care*. London: Longman.

Dockar-Drysdale, B. (1990). *The provision of primary experience: Winnicottian work with children and adolescents*. London: Longman.

Dodge, K. A., & Newman, J. P. (1981). Biased decision-making processes in aggressive boys. *Journal of Abnormal Psychology, 90*, 375–379.

Durkheim, E. ([1893]/1964). *The division of labour in society*. New York: Free Press.

Durkheim, E. ([1897]/1952). *Suicide*. London and New York: Routledge and Keegan Paul.

Eisner, M. (2014). From swords to words: Does macro-level change in self-control predict long-term variation in levels of homicide? In M Tonry (Ed.). *Why crime rates fall and why they don't* (*crime and justice: a review of research*, Vol. 43 Edited by Michael Tonry). Chicago and London: University f Chicago Press.

Eysenck, H. J. (1977). *Crime and personality* (3rd ed.). London: Routledge and Keegan Paul.

Eysenck, S. B. G., & Eysenck, H. J. (1971). Crime and personality: Item analysis of questionnaire responses. *British Journal of Criminology, 11*, 49–62.

Eysenck, S. B. G., & McGurk, B. J. (1980). Impulsiveness and venturesomeness in a detention centre population. *Psychological Reports, 47*, 1299–1306.

Farrell, M. (1984). Professor eysenck's theory of crime: A brief explanation. *The Police Journal, 57*(3), 257–261.

Farrell, M. (1988a). Testing the eysenck theory. *Police Review, 96*(4949), 382–383.

Farrell, M. (1988b). What rocky got out of differential association. *The Criminologist, 12*(4), 236–237.

Farrell, M. (1989). Positivism and crime. *The Criminologist, 13*(4), 220–221.

Farrell, M. (1990). The 'new' criminology. *The Criminologist, 14*(1), 46–47.

Farrell, M. (1991). Strain theory. *The Criminologist, 15*(2), 107–108.

Felson, M. (1994). *Crime and everyday life*. Newbury Park, CA: Pine Forge Press.

Farrell, M. (2012). *New perspectives in special education: Contemporary philosophical debates*. New York and London: Routledge.

Ferracuti, F., & Wolfgang, M. E. ([1967]/2010). *The subculture of violence: Towards an integrated theory in criminology*. London and New York: Routledge.
Fishbein, D. H. (1996). The biology of antisocial behaviour. In J. E. Conklin (Ed.). *New perspectives in criminology*. Boston, MA: Allyn and Bacon.
Freud, S. ([1920]/2001). Beyond the pleasure principle. In *Beyond the pleasure principle, group psychology and other Works*. The standard edition of the complete psychological works of sigmund freud, Vol. 18, 1920–1922 (Translated from the German under the general editorship of James Strachey) pp. 7-66 London, Vintage The Hogarth Press and the Institute of Psychoanalysis.
Freud, S. ([1927]/2001). The future of an illusion. In *The future of an illusion, civilisation and its discontents and other works*. The Standard Edition of the Complete Psychological Works of Sigmund Freud, Vol. 21, 1927–1931 (Translated from the German under the general editorship of James Strachey) pp. 1–56. London, Vintage: The Hogarth Press and the Institute of Psychoanalysis.
Gelsthorpe, L., & Morriss, A. (1988). Feminism and criminology in Britain. *British Journal of Criminology, 28*(2), 93–110.
Hirschi, T. (1969). *The causes of delinquency Berkley*. CA: University of California Press.
Hollin, C. R. (2012). Criminological psychology. In M. Maguire, R. Morgan, & R. Reiner (Eds.), *The Oxford handbook of criminology* (5th ed.). Oxford: Oxford University Press.
Hollin, C. L., & Wheeler, H. M. (1982). The violent young offender: A small group study of a borstal population. *Journal of Adolescence, 5*, 247–257.
Hough, R. M., & McCorkle, K. D. (2017). *American homicide*. Thousand Oaks, CA and London: Sage.
Husserl, E. ([1913a]/1980). *Ideas pertaining to a pure phenomenology and to a phenomenological philosophy, third book: Phenomenology and the foundations of science* (Translated from the German by R. Rojcewitz and A. Schuwer) Dordrecht, Kluwer.
Husserl, E. ([1913b]/1982). *Ideas pertaining to a pure phenomenology and to a phenomenological philosophy, first book: General introduction to a pure phenomenology* (Translated from the German by R. Rojcewitz and A. Schuwer) Dordrecht: Kluwer.
Husserl, E. ([1913c]/1989). *Ideas pertaining to a pure phenomenology and to a phenomenological philosophy, second book: Studies in the phenomenology of constitution* (Translated from the German by R. Rojcewitz and A. Schuwer) Dordrecht: Kluwer.
Jeffrey, C. R. (1965). Criminal behaviour and learning theory. *Journal of Criminal Law, Criminology and Police Science, 56*, 294–300.
Kohlberg, L. (1978). Revisions in the theory and practice of mental development. In Damon, W. (Ed.), *New directions in child development: Moral development*. San Francisco, CA, Jessey-Bass.
Laub, J., & Sampson, R. (2003). *Shared beginnings divergent lives: Delinquent boys to age 70 Cambridge*. Mass: Harvard University Press.
Lukes, S. (1967). Alienation and anomie. In P. Laslett & W. Runciman (Eds.). *Philosophy, politics and society*. Oxford: Blackwell.
Maguire, M., Morgan, R., & Reiner, R. (2012). *The Oxford handbook of criminology* (5th ed.). Oxford: Oxford University Press.
McGurk, B. J., & McDougal, C. (1981). A new approach to eysenck's theory of criminality. *Personality and Individual Differences, 2*, 338–340.
Mednick, S. A., Moffitt, T. E., & Stack, S. (Eds.). (1987). *The causes of crime: New biological approaches*. Cambridge: Cambridge University Press.
Merton, R. K. (1938). Social structure and anomie. *American Sociological Review, 3*, 672–682.
Monkton-Smith, J. (2012). *Murder, gender and the media: Narratives of dangerous love*. Basingstoke UK: Palgrave Macmillan.
Nagy, V. A. (2015). *Nineteenth century female poisoners: thee english women who used arsenic to kill*. Basingstoke UK: Palgrave Macmillan.
Palmer, E. J. (2003). *Offending behaviour: Moral reasoning, criminal conduct and rehabilitation of offenders*. Cullompton, Devon: Willan Publishing.

Park, R. (1925). Community organisation and juvenile delinquency. In R. Park & R. Burgess (Eds.), *The city Chicago*. ILL: University of Chicago Press.

Raine, A., Buchsbaum, M., & LaCasse, L. (1997). Brain abnormalities in murderers indicated by positron emission tomography. *Biological Psychiatry, 42*(6), 495–508.

Raine, A., Buchsbaum, M., Stanely, J., Lottenberg, S., Abel, L., & Stoddard, J. (1994). Selective reductions in prefrontal glucose metabolism in murderers assessed with positron emission tomography. *Biological Psychiatry, 36*(1), 365–373.

Rock, P. (2012). Sociological theories of crime. In M. Maguire, R. Morgan, & R. Reiner (Eds.), *The Oxford handbook of criminology* (5th ed., 39–80). Oxford: Oxford University Press.

Rotter, J. B. (1966). Generalised expectancies for internal versus external control of reinforcement. *Psychological Monographs: General and Applied, 80*(1), (Whole Number 69).

Seal, L. (2010). *Women, murder and femininity: Gender representations of women who kill*. Basingstoke, UK: Palgrave Macmillan.

Shaw, C. (1971). Male Juvenile Delinquency and group behaviour. In J. Short (Ed.), *The social fabric of the metropolis Chicago*. ILL: University of Chicago Press.

Sherman, L., Gartin, P., & Buerger, M. (1989, February). Hot spots of predatory crime: Routine activities and the criminology of place. *Criminology, 27*(1), 27–56.

Skinner, B. F. (1938). *The behaviour of organisms: An experimental analysis*. New York: Appleton-Century-Crofts.

Slaby, R. G., & Guerra, N. G. (1988). Cognitive mediators of aggression in adolescent offenders: 1, assessment. *Developmental Psychology, 24,* 580–588.

Snider, L. (1998). Towards safer societies: Punishment, masculinities and violence against women. *British Journal of Criminology, 38*(1), 1–39.

Spierenburg, P. (2008). *A history of murder: Personal violence in Europe from the middle ages to the present*. Cambridge: Polity Press.

Sutherland, E. H. (1947). *Principles of criminology* (2nd ed.). Philadelphia, PA: Lippincott.

Taylor, I., Walton, P., & Young, J. (1973). *The new criminology: For a social theory of deviancy*. London, Routledge and Keegan Paul.

Walklate, S. (2001). *Gender crime and criminal justice*. UK, Willan: Cullompton.

Watson, K. (2004). *Poisoned lives: English Poisoners and their victims*. London and New York: Hambledon and London.

Williams, K. (2001). *Textbook on criminology*. London: Blackstone.

Young, J. (1997). Left realist criminology. In M. Maguire, R. Morgan, & and R. Reiner. (Eds.). *The Oxford handbook of criminology* (2nd ed.). Oxford: Oxford University Press.

Chapter 4
Understanding Poisons

Introduction

Before looking at the nature of poisons, it will be useful to consider how people's general interest in noxious substances has developed and persisted over time. Having set the scene in this way, we then tackle how to define poison. Classifications of poisons (such as plant, animal, elemental) further inform the picture. Ways of describing the characteristics of poisons (for example colour, odour and taste) help to identify particular ones. Other issues concern the use of poisons in homicide. Characteristics of some toxic substances can make them less likely to be detected. Comparisons and contrasts can be made between poisoning and homicide using other means such as firearms. Also important are different ways in which poisons are administered, how they act on the human body, and how fatal dose is represented. Acute and chronic poisoning can be usefully distinguished. Modern day antidotes and the treatment of poisoning require understanding. One can also make judgements about possible future trends in homicidal poisoning.

Poisons and Poisoning in the Past

As Thompson ([1931]/1993) speculates, early humans in their search for, 'curative substances' no doubt came across 'noxious ones' (Ibid. p. 12). Such substances from plant juices and perhaps snake venom would have constituted the early arrow poisons which were used in remote parts of the world into the twentieth century (Farrell 1995). If in early human groups, certain individuals remembered certain plants and perhaps insects and grubs that when consumed would cause stupor or death, they would likely accrue power and influence.

In tradition, legend and mythology, poisons regularly arise. Revered by the Sumerians, the Goddess Ninisina (or Gula) was associated with toxins, being also

M. Farrell, *Criminology of Homicidal Poisoning*,
DOI 10.1007/978-3-319-59117-9_4

called among her many names, 'controller of noxious poisons' (Hayes and Gilbert 2009, p. 4).

From Egypt, the Ebers papyrus (1500 B.C.E.) mentions more than 700 substances and over 300 recipes which refer to poisonous or medicinal plants and minerals. These include opium, hemlock, aconite, lead and antimony. Ancient Egyptians according to this source mixed poppy opium, pepper and fragrant spices in wine.

Persians in ancient times are said to have studied poisoning. Plutarch reports a suspicion that Queen Parysatis during the reign of Artaxerxes II (405-359 B.C.E.) poisoned her daughter in law Queen Statira. She used a knife one side of whose blade had been coated with venom. A game bird set before the two diners was carved carefully with the prepared implement so that Parysatis could eat safely while Statira soon after died (Thompson [1931]/1993, p. 30).

Mithridates (132-63 B.C.E.) King of Pontus in Asia Minor experimented with poisons. His efforts to develop a universal antidote came to be known a 'Mithridates' or 'Mithridaticum' and contained many ingredients including viper flesh.

Minerals such as arsenic and plants with poisonous properties were known in India in centuries past. Many early Sanskrit manuscripts were prepared with orpiment (arsenic) to preserve them from attacks by insects. Among the noxious plants known in India is aconite of which various species are common. It is thought that this was originally used as an arrow poison. Both roots and leaves of the Indian Oleander (*nerium odorum*) contain a poison principle affecting the heart. The root of the climbing lily (*gloriosa superba*) can yield a poisonous alkaloid related to colchicine (Thompson ([1931]/1993, p. 32).

In China, the Chou ritual said to date from 246 B.C.E. provides an account of state medical services comprising five departments. Medicaments used by the group included the 'five poisons' which appear to have included cinnabar (mercury), realgar (arsenic) and green vitriol (copper sulphate). From great antiquity, the Chinese are said to have employed gold leaf for suicidal purposes, placing it over the lips and then rapidly inhaling so that it passes into the throat, blocking the glottis and causing suffocation (Thompson ([1931]/1993, p. 33).

Ancient Greeks knew of arsenic in the form of realgar (an arsenic sulphide mineral which owing to its red-orange colour is sometime known as 'ruby of arsenic') and orpiment (another arsenic sulphide which is rich yellow in colour). They also knew of antimony, lead, mercury and copper. Hemlock appears to have been the chief vegetable poison used by the Greeks. In fact, the state poison was mainly composed of a species of hemlock known as cicuta (Thompson [1931]/1993, p. 23). Theophrastus of Eresus (circa 372-287 B.C.E.) the philosopher and writer on botany, cites poison extracted from wolf's bane (aconite) and mentions the erroneous belief that there were 'time' or 'slow' poisons capable of having their effect months or even years after being consumed (see also Farrell 1997a).

Regarding ancient Rome, it is difficult to separate poison rumour from poison fact. For example, Livy (59 B.C.E.–17 A.D.) states that in a few years before 203 B.C.E. a series of poisonings were perpetrated by a Roman noblewoman, the deaths having been attributed to plague. A female slave then informed the soldier and consul Quintus Verrucosus (d. 203 B.C.E.) that the dead had been poisoned and accordingly, twenty suspects were seized by the officers of justice. Claiming that they had only been involved in preparing medicinal drugs, the suspects agreed to a request to take their own concoctions as proof of this. All of them reputedly died as a result (see also, Farrell 1996).

In Italy in the early seventeenth century, Naples was a centre of poisoning knowledge and practice. A certain 'Toffana' is said to have been responsible for many murders often by selling arsenic in solution to those who planned a poisoning. Tortured on the rack, she confessed to her crimes (Thompson [1931]/1993, pp. 144–147). Cesare Borgia, son of Pope Alexander 6th was rumoured to have poisoned opponents on behalf of the Pontiff. Among victims were thought to be the Duke of Grandier. Cesare Borgia was reputed to have a secret room where he mixed his poisons and which no one was permitted to enter except the Pope himself, and Cesare's sister Lucretia (Ibid.).

Florentine Catherine de' Medici who married King Henry II is reputed to have brought the skills of poisoning from Italy to France. A well-known seventeenth century case from France is that of the Marquise de Brinvilliers (1630–1676). Having poisoned her father and two brothers she was tried and executed by decapitation with a sword.

In the glossary to this book, are referenced over 100 cases of poisoning from the nineteenth century to the present day. It is these more recent cases that are mainly the subject of discussion throughout the book, used to illustrate various points about poisons and poisoners, their victims and other circumstances of such homicides.

Defining Poison

One begins with confidence when facing the task of defining poison. Everyone has an idea of what is a poison. It is clear that a poison is able to kill or to do harm to a person. Examples can readily be given such as arsenic, strychnine or cyanide. However, when one looks in more detail at the challenge, initial confidence begins to be tested and it soon emerges that the concept is slippery (Farrell 1990).

Poisoning is not necessarily intrinsic to a substance but can vary with the amount consumed. Morphine is an example, being beneficial in small doses (as when used to control pain) but lethal in larger quantities. It is a maxim of toxicology that 'the dose makes the poison' (Kolok 2016, pp. 1–9). Despite this, we can still say that poisons generally have a harmful effect in small amounts. Even when considering lethal doses of morphine, one is still dealing with tiny quantities. To take a further example of arsenic, a teaspoonful is several times the typical lethal dose.

Confusingly, in the past, some poisons were mistakenly thought to have beneficial effects in very small quantities. Peasants in the province of Styria (a state in southern Austria) thought that arsenic improved the 'wind' for climbing hills (Christie 1968). Into the 1950s, medicinal uses of arsenic included the treatment of leukaemia and its deployment as an external paste for carious teeth. Also, well into the twentieth century, arsenic was erroneously imbibed for its supposed tonic effects. Gradually, caution became more widespread and the outcomes were recognised as 'unpredictable and uncontrollable' (Martindale 1958). In more recent times, practically the only therapeutic use of arsenic was that of Melarsoprol in treating the tropical disease trypanosomiasis (sleeping sickness).

Certain substances having a harmful effect are not deemed toxic. Boiling liquids would injure the body but, because their effect depends on temperature, they are not considered poisons. Powdered glass if swallowed certainly injures but because its action is 'mechanical' it too is excluded from any definition. Allergies can create in those affected harmful responses to substances (for example pollen or nuts) that to others are benign, so that the substances of themselves cannot be considered as poisons.

An immediate assumption when thinking of poisons is that they are taken by mouth, but of course, poisons can be absorbed into the body in other ways, for example by being injected into the bloodstream or under the skin.

Bringing these points together begins to point towards a suitable definition. A poison must be able to kill or do serious harm to the functioning of bodily organs or tissues. Secondly, it has its effect in small doses. The substance must not be dependent on mechanical action or temperature, or individual bodily peculiarities for its effect. Different poisons (or the same poison in different forms) may be introduced to the body in different ways.

Over the years, acceptable definitions have incorporated some if not all of these points. For Genaro (1979) a poison is, 'A substance that in relatively small doses, has an action, when it is ingested by, injected into, inhaled or absorbed by, or applied to a living organism, that either destroys life or impairs seriously the functions of one or more organs or tissues'. In the 31st edition of *Dorland's Illustrated Medical Dictionary* (Anderson 2007) poison is stated to be, 'any substance that, when relatively small amounts are ingested, inhaled, or absorbed, or applied to, injected into, or developed within the body, has chemical action that causes damage to structure, or disturbance of function, producing symptoms, illness or death'. As an indication of a settled brief definition, the same dictionary under its founder (Dorland 1985) offered a very similar delineation over twenty years previously although without reference to the fact that poison may produce 'symptoms, illness or death'.

Classifications of Poisons

Poisons can be classified in many ways. For example, attempts are made to group them according to their source as being organic or inorganic. Organic poisons include plant poisons like digitalis; animal poisons such as cantharides; bacterial poisons for example diphtheria, and certain synthetic compounds such as chloroform, synthetic drugs such as Seconal sodium and succinylcholine chloride; and the contact herbicide Paraquat. Also included would be cyanides (salts of cyanic acid). Turning to inorganic poisons these include elements and their salts, notably arsenic, copper, lead, mercury and antimony as well as phosphorus and thallium.

In looking at poisons that have been used for murder, I make a slightly different grouping which recognises plant, animal and bacterial poisons, but which groups recognised medicinal drugs separately, brings together elements and their derivatives and compounds (including organic ones) and brings together a few 'other poisons' separately. As with any other grouping this has areas of overlap. For example it classes morphine as a plant poison when it is also considered to be a medical drug.

As explained, poisons considered here are grouped, for convenience and to hopefully help exposition under several headings:

- Plants poisons: colchicum seeds; atropine (belladonna) ; aconite; strychnine; opium and morphine; cyanide, potassium cyanide and prussic acid; digitalis; nicotine; hyoscine.
- Animal poisons: Cantharides, insulin.
- Bacterial poisons: typhoid, tuberculosis, diphtheria.
- Drugs: Fentanyl; Methylphenobarbitone; Seconal sodium; succinylcholine chloride, Vecuronium bromide.
- Elements, their compounds and derivatives: Arsenic; antimony and tartar emetic; copper; phosphorus; organic phosphorus compound E605; lead; mercuric chloride; thallium; potassium chloride.
- Other poisons: carbon monoxide; chloroform; nitric acid, hydrochloric acid; Paraquat; anti-freeze; *N*-Nitrosodimethylamine.

In the present book, plant, animal and bacterial poisons and drugs and the homicidal cases involving them are discussed in Chap. 5. Elements and 'other poisons' are similarly treated in Chap. 6.

Ways of Describing Characteristics of Poisons

Convenient and systematic ways of describing poisons tend to be used. These include specifying the type of poison (such as whether it is an element, plant or bacteria) and its different forms where this is relevant. Reference may be made to the chemical structure of the substance. Also pertinent are colour, odour and taste or lack of them. Where the substance has or had a regular legitimate use this is described. It is important to know how the body absorbs the substance (for example through the gastrointestinal tract), how it is distributed in the body, and how it is excreted. Whatever action the poison has on the human body is described. Symptoms are detailed and it may be specified which ones tend to appear early or late in the course of the poison's action. Typical lethal dose is often cited. Sometimes, the treatment or antidote for the poison may be noted.

To briefly sketch out an example, arsenic is an elemental semi-metal whose compounds are highly poisonous. The form in which it has often been used as a homicidal poison is its inorganic trivalent structure (having three electrons available for bonding with other substances) of arsenic trioxide (white arsenic). This looks like sugar, and is almost tasteless. White arsenic has been used as a rodent poison, in insecticides and herbicides, and in the textile, glass and enamel industries. Because arsenic trioxide is absorbed only slowly in water, the rate at which the body absorbs it depends on how finely it has been powdered, how it is administered, how much has been consumed, and over what period of time. Arsenic is predominantly stored in heart, lung, liver and kidney tissue and is excreted mainly but not solely in urine. Regarding action, trivalent arsenicals primarily binds to sulphur atoms in the body's enzymes. They inhibit syphydril containing enzyme systems essential to normal cellular metabolism. Symptoms of acute and chronic arsenic poisoning differ. Just to take the example of acute symptoms, these can include burning lips, tightening of the throat and difficulty swallowing, followed by severe gastric pains, violent vomiting, and excessive watery diarrhoea, raging thirst and muscular craps. As fluid is lost through vomiting and diarrhoea, symptoms of 'shock' appear. Coma and death follow. The minimal recorded lethal dose of arsenic is about one grain.

Features of Less Detectable Poisons

Certain characteristics of some poisons can, all other things being equal, render them less likely to be detected. For example, unlike some other modus operandi, poisons are not obvious at the crime scene as are bullet wounds or stab wounds, so it may not be apparent that a crime has been committed at all. If a poison is administered in bland food and has a bitter taste, it is more likely to be noticed by the victim than a tasteless, odourless poison given with the same meal. Should a poison be easily soluble in water, it is more likely to be dissolved and go undetected in food or drink.

An estimate of the time that a poison takes to act has to be built into the plan that the poisoner has for killing. The more unusual the poison, the less likely (it might be thought) that it will be detected, but this is not always the case. However exotic the poison if it is clear that poisoning has taken place, the chance of detection is increased. Where a poison is easy to obtain, the less likely it is to be traced to the perpetrator. So for example where a poison can be obtained naturally from a plant, it can be harder to trace than one that has to be purchased and signed for. If a poison is found naturally in a place of burial as is arsenic, it is more difficult to prove that the substance was administered before death and was not simply absorbed into the body from grave earth.

Should a poison mimic the symptoms of a disease or condition that is prevalent in a particular country at a certain time it may go unnoticed. Symptoms of arsenic poisoning have been mistaken for sunstroke and cholera.

Poison Homicide and Other Homicides

Some characteristics of poison murder can be teased out by comparing and contrasting them to other modus operandi. Murder by stabbing involves the victim usually being fully aware that harm is intended and perhaps having the opportunity to call for help or to take defensive action. With poisoning, the victim may not be aware that they are being killed and therefore be unable to mount any defence.

Stabbing will leave a wound, making it quickly clear that a killing has taken place. By contrast poison homicide need not lead a wound (although the injection of a poison will leave a tiny puncture) and it may not be apparent that murder has occurred. Stabbing is unlikely to be inadvertent but murder by poisoning can be made to look accidental by the perpetrator suggesting that the victim took an accidental overdose of a drug.

Administration of Poisons

Poison can be given orally, concealed in food, drink, or medicine. It may be administered by injection under the skin or into the bloodstream perhaps under the pretext of administering a medication. Unusually, in Guandong Province, China, soup laced with sleeping pills and dichlorvos (insecticide) was injected directly into the stomach by a carer He Tiandai [101] to poison her elderly client He Yanzhu.

Children have been poisoned by introducing a harmful substance through a feeding tube. As a gas or fine powder, poison can be inhaled into the lungs and so enter the blood stream. Some poisons can be absorbed from contact with the skin surface. Highly unusually, poisoning death can be caused by rectal enema or by vaginal pessary. In 2007 Tammy Jane Warner of Lake Jackson, US was accused of negligent homicide in administering a sherry enema to her alcoholic husband who because of throat problems could not drink alcohol—the case was dropped for lack of evidence (Stewart 2007). Death by poison has been caused (negligently) by vaginal pessary for example by using arsenic on a pessary stick as an abortifacient (Karmakar 2015, p. 86).

Action of Poisons

Action on Enzymes

One of the ways in which poisons act is by attacking enzymes, the protein molecules that bring about chemical reactions in other substances (Anderson 2007, p. 635). Found in many body tissues and in digestive fluids, many hundreds of enzymes have been identified. Although produced by living cells, enzymes operate independently as catalysts. Being essential to the proper functioning of the body, enzymes can in small amounts, effect large scale transformations of various compounds. Each enzyme has a specialised function and affects a particular chemical reaction in the body. While some enzymes are present in large amounts, others occur in comparatively small quantities. Some are not so important while others are 'key' enzymes. Being delicate, they are easily destroyed for example by heat. Acids and alkalis destroy them because enzymes are active only within a certain range of acidity or alkalinity. Structured as a complex network of atoms of hydrogen, carbon, oxygen, nitrogen, sulphur and others, enzymes may be globular or have loops and twists that are easily destroyed by poison.

When a poison inhibits enzyme activity, this can cause enormous damage. Clearly, if a poison attacks an enzyme which is both a key enzyme and is present only in relatively small amounts, this is particularly destructive. If enough molecules of a poison are present, an enzyme can be destroyed. Among poisons affecting enzymes are cyanide, lead, arsenic and antimony. Cyanide for example attacks an enzyme in the blood. Some poisons attack enzymes in the nervous system and consequently a distinction between poisons attacking enzymes and those affecting the nervous system is not absolutely rigid but can still be useful.

Poisons Influencing the Nervous System

Poisons affecting the central nervous system (brain and spinal cord) may depress or stimulate it. Among drugs depressing the central nervous system are barbiturates, for example Seconal sodium which in too large a dose causes death by this depressant action. By contrast, strychnine stimulates the central nervous system although it acts in other ways too.

Turning to the peripheral nervous system, this comprises the somatic and autonomic systems. The somatic system is responsible for carrying motor and sensory information to and from the central nervous system. It activates voluntary muscles via a nerve-muscle junction between the motor nerve and the muscle end plate. This junction is essentially a 'gap' alternately filled by a fluid that allows the nerve impulse to pass, and one that destroys the first fluid. An impulse travelling down the nerve releases some of the clusters of acetylcholine which are stored at nerve endings, allowing the acetylcholine to bridge the gap and touch the membrane on the other side. At rest, this membrane is 'polarised' with a negative electrical charge on the inside and a positive charge on the outside. Acetylcholine changes the membrane's electrical condition (depolarises it), sending an impulse to the muscle. To prevent continual stimulation of the muscle, the second fluid, cholinesterase, is released destroying the acetylcholine and breaking the connection. This whole process takes only a five hundredth of a second.

Curare-based drugs compete with the acetylcholine. Combining with the receptors on the muscle end plate and blocking them, these drugs prevent the end plate from being depolarised by the acetylcholine, weakening and paralysing the muscles. Other substances act by depolarisation. Succinylcholine chloride for example, mimics the action of acetylcholine at the motor end plate causing the voluntary muscles to contract. Unlike acetylcholine however, the drug is not destroyed straight away, so depolarisation continues. However, this does not lead to continued muscle contraction. This may be because the drug simultaneously decreases the excitability of the end plate and the muscular block may be as much owing to this as to depolarisation. Indeed the two effects may be interrelated.

Other poisons work on the autonomic nervous system which is concerned with internal organs, blood vessels and so called secreting glands, and functions mainly independently of the will. Comprising ganglia (nerve cell clusters) connected by nerve fibres, the system is situated in the neck, chest and abdomen, and consists of a sympathetic and a parasympathetic system. While the sympathetic system augments heart action and inhibits intestine action, the parasympathetic system (connected with the central nervous system through nerve centres in the mid brain medulla and lower end of the spinal cord) inhibits heart action and augments intestine action. Nerve cells transmit or receive nerve impulses. Outgoing impulses are conveyed by efferent nerves to muscles and blood vessels, while incoming impulses are conveyed to the nerve cells by afferent nerves carrying messages from sense organs, skins, joints and so on. Acetylcholine is again important because, as in the parasympathetic system, it transmits nerve impulses to the brain. It mediates transmission from nerve to nerve and from nerve to organs. Atropine is a poison that disturbs the parasympathetic system by blocking the effect of acetylcholine.

Corrosives, Irritants and Narcotics

As well as the classifications of poisons according to their action on enzymes or on the nervous system, poisons can be grouped according to their mode of action, for example whether they are corrosive, irritant or narcotic.

Corrosive poisons burn and destroy tissue on contact, acting directly. Corrosive poisons include strong mineral acids such as nitric acid; alkalis such as caustic soda (sodium hydroxide or lye), or ammonia; and certain strong salts, for example corrosive sublimate.

Irritant poisons produce inflammation or irritation often in the stomach and intestines. They can cause vomiting, diarrhoea and abdominal pain, collapse, unconsciousness and death. Among irritants are white arsenic (arsenious acid), yellow arsenic (orpiment), acetate of lead, sulphate of copper, subacetate of copper, arsenate of copper (Scheele's Green), tartrated antimony (tartar emetic) and phosphorus.

Narcotics affect the central nervous system causing stupor. Substances that are predominantly narcotic include opium and its derivatives, prussic acid (hydrocyanic acid), potassium cyanide and chloroform. Poisonous gases such as carbon monoxide are also included as narcotics. Generally speaking, the symptoms produced by narcotic poisoning include headache, giddiness, visual problems, stupor, unconsciousness, coma and ultimately death.

Many narcotics also have an irritant effect and are further classified as narcotic-irritants (or acronarcotics) which comprise substances causing symptoms or irritation such as sickness, vomiting, convulsions, delirium or excitement. Examples associated with plants are strychnine (nux vomica), foxglove (Digitalis purpurea), monk's hood (Aconitum napelus), henbane (Hyoscyamus niger), deadly nightshade (Atropa belladonna), tobacco (Nicotiana tabacum), spotted hemlock (Conium maculatum) and some types of poisonous fungi. Symptoms begin with vomiting, diarrhoea and stomach pains, and progress to delirium and convulsions, stupor and eventually death.

Fatal Dose and How It Is Represented

Just as it at first seems straightforward to define poisons, although in practice it is not so easy, so it appears that fatal dose could be stated straightforwardly, whereas in fact this is quite difficult. Many factors influence the outcome of poisoning. For the victim, their age, gender, prior physical health and emotional health all play a part.

Previous exposure to the poison concerned is influential. In some instances of chronic arsenic poisoning, the doses appear to have had a cumulative effect leading slowly to death. Sometimes it seems hardly conceivable that death did not occur following a particular poison dose. In the plot to murder Russian faith healer Rasputin (through the involvement of Prince Youssoupov) he was first given cakes liberally sprinkled with cyanide and Madeira wine similarly poisoned. His breathing became laboured, but a further glass of poisoned wine seemed only to revive him. The mystic was then shot, following which he was thrown into the river Neva (Farrell 1997b, 1998).

How a poison is distributed by the body after it has been administered is relevant. Some 'latch onto' blood, some to nerve tissues, some to proteins. Water soluble poisons tend to have difficulty reaching the central nervous system because of the blood–brain barrier of fatty substances around the capillaries of the nervous system which tends to repel water and consequently deter any water-borne material.

Method of ingestion of a poison is influential, for example, whether it is swallowed, inhaled as gas or fumes, absorbed through the skin surface, or injected in skin or into blood vessels.

It will be clear that the question, 'What is the lethal dose of poison X?' is a complex one which cannot always be answered accurately. Attempts are made however. A fatal dose of a poison is usually expressed in terms of its weight. About

100 mg. of strychnine taken orally represents a fatal dose, the minimum lethal dose being some 36 mg. A fatal dose of methanol (a very large component of gas-line antifreeze) is about 20–150 gm.

Fatal dose may be specified according to the amount that is likely to cause death according to whether the victim is an adult or a child. For the plant poison atropine, death has been reported after doses of less than 10 mg for children and smaller than 100 mg for adults. An indication of a lethal amount may be conveyed in relation to the victim's body weight. A minimum lethal dose of cyanide is estimated to be between 0.7 and 3.5 mg per kilo of body weight making a possible lethal dose of 200 mg about the weight of four postage stamps. For an adult, the minimum lethal dose of thallium sulphate is about 800 mg. For a person weighing 70 kg, this is 12 mg per kg of body weight.

Vivid comparisons may be made to convey the toxicity of some poisons. For arsenic, the minimal recorded lethal dose is about 200 mg making a teaspoon of the substance is about seven times this amount. By contrast, copper sulphate is in relative terms *not* one of the most toxic poisons, some 10 g being a possible lethal quantity.

One attempt to standardise lethal doses is to record the percentages of deaths in animals that have been administered the poison in question. Hence, the minimum lethal dose is that for which a fatality has been recorded. Accordingly, LD50 means that a poison in a specified amount constituted a lethal dose in 50% of the animals tested while LD100 is the dose at which all the test population were killed. To give an idea of the relative lethal dose of certain poisons, it can be noted that the lethal dose of thallium is about five times greater than that of cyanide or arsenic (Trestrail 2007, p. 38).

Acute and Chronic Poisoning

In a medical context, one might speak of the acute effects of poisoning as the immediate ones and refer to the chronic effects as those that occur later from the same poisons. With reference to homicide, an acute poisoning is intended to kill the victim quickly while chronic poisoning kills slowly over a longer period. Sometimes poisoners use a combination of chronic poisoning perhaps to suggest a lingering illness followed by acute poisoning to secure death. It is not always possible to say that a particular poison acts acutely or chronically because this depends on such factors as the dose and the form in which the poison is administered (orally, intravenously and so on).

As already indicated, regarding arsenic, the same poison can be administered to kill a victim while producing acute symptoms or chronic symptoms. Poisoners may choose acute or chronic poisoning according to their intentions and motivation as will be discussed further in a later chapter on 'Poisoners and their characteristics'.

Antidotes and Treatment for Poisoning

Briefly defined, an antidote is, 'a remedy for counteracting a poison' (Anderson 2007, p. 104).

A chemical antidote, as its name suggests, reacts chemically with a poison to form a harmless compound. Some antidotes act 'mechanically' to stop a poison from being absorbed. A physiologic antidote produces opposing effects to those caused by the poison concerned, so counteracting it. Antidotes and the vain search for a universal antidote that would be effective for any poison have their origins in folklore, superstition and ancient history (Farrell 1992, pp. 17–19).

A modern day general antidote for poisons is activated charcoal (Olsen 2010). It is made by the controlled heating of burned wood, peat or similar substances at 540 °C in an atmosphere of air, water vapour or carbon dioxide. This creates numerous minute pores to form in the charcoal which can absorb liquids, gases or substances dissolved in fluids. Parisian pharmacist P.F. Touery provided a memorable demonstration of the effectiveness of activated charcoal before the French Academy in 1830. After swallowing ten times the fatal dose of strychnine, he immediately consumed 15 g of activated charcoal and was unharmed. Activated charcoal is not effective for all poisons, being powerless for example against cyanide. But it can absorb to take just some examples, arsenic, digitalis, morphine, nicotine, opium, phosphorus, and, mercifully for Touery, strychnine. Even when some poisons have been taken up by the bloodstream, activated charcoal can still be used to absorb them as when blood is passed through a B-D Hemodetoxifier, an instrument that soaks up the poison before the blood is pumped back into the body.

Possible Trends in Poisoning

Attempts have been made to ascertain any trends in the use of particular poisons. From a database of 1026 cases in which the offender was convicted of homicidal poisoning, and extending chronologically from before the Christian era to the present day, Trestrail (2007) identified the most commonly used poisons as arsenic (26% of cases), cyanide (8%) and strychnine (6%), these three totalling 40% of poisons used.

Watson (2004) analysed assize records and other sources concerning criminal poisoning cases from 1750 to 1914 showing the poisons that were used in English criminal cases. Of the 332 inorganic poisons the most common were arsenic (237), mercury (32) and acids—hydrochloric, sulphuric and nitric (24). Regarding organic poisons, 172 were used, with the most common being opium and laudanum (52) strychnine and nux vomica (41) and acids—acetic, carbolic, oxalic, tartaric and prussic including cyanides (34) (Ibid. p. 33 Table 1).

Suggesting possible trends in poisonings, a study looked at the number of homicidal poisonings and the methods used in several places: Sweden, and several parts of the United States (Miami-Dade County, Florida; New York City, NY; Oakland County, Michigan). The researchers concluded that poisoning is an 'infrequently established crime'. Carefully chosen, the phrase shows that the writers recognise that the symptoms and signs of poison victims can often be misdiagnosed as natural disease, especially in a hospital setting. Accordingly, the authors recognise that 'an unknown number of homicides go undetected'. In the cases that were examined, the chosen poison appears to have changed over time. In the past, frequently used poisons included arsenic, cyanide and parathion (an organic phosphorus compound was also known as E605). In the present day the researchers found, that narcotics (often derived from opium or similar) are more commonly detected in poison victims (Finneberg et al. 2013).

In line with the finding that drugs were more commonly used in poisonings, Shepherd and Ferlew (2009) looked at homicidal poisoning deaths in the US, interrogating the National Mortality Statistics database for the years 1999–2005 and analysing some 523 homicidal poisoning deaths. They found that medications were the most common poison.

Trends in the use of particular poisons are likely to relate to access to specific poisons and to people's knowledge of them. In the nineteenth century (and perhaps the early twentieth century) rural folkloric knowledge of plants and their healing as well as their harmful properties made poisonous plants a possible choice for homicide. Easy availability of substances such as arsenic before legislation began to tighten access again made it a possible choice. (It was also comparatively cheap). In more recent times, drugs have been developed and are taken by large numbers of the population. Easy access to these and the potential to give someone a lethal dose of a drug that they are already taking becomes a possibility not just in medic-patient murders but more widely.

Also the types of poisons that are more readily available have changed over time. Arsenic is no longer an everyday substance, but anti-freeze is, and accordingly instances of its use as a poison come to light. As industries and research requirements change, the substances that are available through them alter. Long after hatters had stopped using arsenic, rocket scientists used potentially lethal *N*-Nitrosodimethylamine. Over-the-counter loopholes may have been addressed, but in recent years poisons have been bought on e-bay or smuggled from other countries where they are more freely available.

Conclusion

Poisons and poisoners can be traced to antiquity and undoubtedly go back to pre-history. Defining a poison is more slippery than at first appears. Classifying poisons (such as plant, animal, bacterial) help systematise the knowledge that we possess about them. Ways of describing the characteristics of poisons help to identify particular ones. Indeed, some qualities such as being odourless and tasteless help make certain poisons, all other things being equal, less likely to be detected. Comparisons and contrasts can be made between murder by poisoning and other modus operandi. For example, whereas it is usually quickly obvious that a victim has been shot, it is not always apparent that someone has been poisoned so that it may not be known that a crime has taken place at all. Poisons can be administered in different ways and they have different ways of acting on the body for example, attacking enzymes, affecting the nervous system, or inflicting damage as corrosives, irritants or narcotics. What is likely to constitute a fatal dose can be represented in several ways and is more complicated than it seems at first. Acute and chronic poisoning may be distinguished. Being aware of modern day antidotes to poisons and more broadly the treatment of poisoning can help fill out basic understanding of poisons. Trends in poisoning can be estimated.

It is apparent that the varied nature of poisons including their different action, symptoms produced, taste, the apparent likelihood of their detection and other features provides a poisoner with a wide range of choices of weapon. Having covered this ground, we are now in a position to look at particular poisons that have been used to perpetrate murder. In the next chapter these comprise plant, animal and bacteriological poisons, and drugs. In the chapter after that, we look at elements and their derivatives and compounds, and at 'other poisons'.

Suggested Activities

Note characteristics of poisons that make them more and less likely to be noticed by the victim to whom they are being administered.

Note the characteristics that, following the death of a victim, might make a poison more and less likely to be detected by police, pathologists and forensic scientists.

Key Texts

Holstege et al. (2010) *Criminal Poisoning: Clinical and Forensic Perspectives* Sudbury, Mass., Jones and Bartlett Publishers

This edited medical text book covers different poisons each in a separate chapter (Chapters 4 through 25 of the 28 chapter book), focusing on the mainly medical diagnostic challenges that are associated with detecting and prosecuting.

References

Anderson, D. M. (2007). *Dorland's illustrated medical dictionary* (31st ed.). Philadelphia, PA: Saunders/Elsevier.

Christie, T. L. (1968). *Etched in arsenic*. London: George G. Harrap.

Dorland, W. A. (1985). *Dorland's illustrated medical dictionary* (26th ed.). Philadelphia, PA: Saunders.

Farrell, M. (1990). What's your poison? *Solicitors Journal, 134*(29), 825.

Farrell, M. (1992) *Poisons and poisoners: An encyclopedia of homicidal poisonings.* London: Robert Hale.

Farrell, M. (1995). Poisons used by primitive tribes. *The Criminologist, 19*(4), 213–218.

Farrell, M. (1996). Homicidal poisonings in ancient Rome. *The Criminologist, 20*(1), 26–28.

Farrell, M. (1997a). Poisons and poisoning in ancient Greece. *The Criminologist, 21*(1), 50–52.

Farrell, M. (1997b). The murder of rasputin. *The Criminologist, 21*(4), 207–214.

Farrell, M. (1998) Poisoned, shot and drowned: Why was rasputin so hard to kill?. *The Criminologist, 22*(4), 235–237 (Winter 1998).

Finneberg, A., Junuzovic, M. & Dragivic et. al (2013). Homicide by poisoning. *American Journal of Forensic Medical Pathology*,34(1), 38–42.

Gennaro, A. R. (1979). *Blakiston's Gould Medical Dictionary* (4th ed.). Blacklick, OH: McGraw Hill.

Hayes, A. N. & Gilbert, S. G. (2009). Historical milestones and discoveries that shaped the toxicology sciences. In A. Luch (Ed.) *Molecular, clinical and environmental toxicology volume 1: Molecular Toxicology*. Basel, Switzerland, and Boston, MA: Birkhäuser Verlag.

Holstege, C.P., Neer, T.M., & Saathoff, G.B., et al. (2010). *Criminal poisoning: clinical and forensic perspectives*. Sudbury, Mass., Jones and Bartlett Publishers.

Karmakar, R. N. (2015). *Forensic medicine and toxicology: Theory, oral and practical* (5th ed.). Kolkata, India: Academic Publishers.

Kolok, A. S. (2016). *Modern poisons: A brief introduction to contemporary toxicology*. Washington, DC: Island Press.

Martindale, W. A. (1958). *The extra pharmacopeia* (24th ed.). London: Pharmaceutical Press.

Olsen, K. R. (2010). Activated charcoal for acute poisoning: One toxicologist's journey. *Journal of Medical Toxicology*, 6, 190–198.

Shepherd, G. & Ferslew, B. C. (2009). Homicidal poisoning deaths in the United States 1999–2005. *Clinical Toxicology*, 47(4), 342–347.

Thompson, C. J. S. ([1931]/1993). *Poisons and poisoners–with historical accounts of famous poison mysteries in ancient and modern times.* London: Barnes and Noble.

Trestrail, J. H. (2007). *Criminal poisoning: Investigational guide for law enforcement, toxicologists, forensic scientists and attorneys* (2nd ed.). Totowa, NJ: Humana Press.

Watson, K. (2004). *Poisoned lives: English poisoners and their victims*. New York, Hambledon and London.

Chapter 5
Poisonous Plants, Animals, Bacteria, and Drugs

Introduction

In the past, local knowledge and rural folklore provided understanding of the toxic (and beneficial) properties of plants enabling them to be used to poison, with sufficient preparation, while the use of animal poisons seems to have been rarer. Bacterial poisons require specialist knowledge to prepare and administer and are rarely used in homicide. By contrast, drug overdoses are more commonly used for homicide because of their widespread legitimate use as medicines and their consequent availability. Furthermore, where individuals do not have legitimate access to drugs, they may be administered in toxic doses after being bought illegally, or stolen.

Plant Poisons (Phytotoxins)

Colchicum Seeds

Colchicum autumnale (*Liliaceae*), more commonly known as autumn crocus or meadow saffron, contains the alkaloid colchine in its flowers, roots, and seeds. This plant or its extract has been used to treat gout, a disorder causing inflammation of the joints and other symptoms connected to an excess of uric acid in the blood. It does this by easing pain and reducing inflammation. The corms (roots) was dried and mixed with alcohol to make a tincture, or used to make wine, liquid extract, dry extract or a mixture. *Colchicum* flowers were dried and used as a tincture, while dried seeds could be used either as a tincture or as a liquid extract. More recently, corm, seed and flower preparations have been replaced by colchine, an alkaloid extract from the plant. This may be administered orally as tablets or intravenously. Colchine has also been used to treat a form of chronic leukaemia.

M. Farrell, *Criminology of Homicidal Poisoning*,
DOI 10.1007/978-3-319-59117-9_5

Colchine inhibits cell division which is related to its anti-inflammatory effect. Symptoms of poisoning include nausea, vomiting, diarrhoea and abdominal pain. Delayed symptoms include seizures, shock, and kidney, liver and respiratory failure. Death may be caused by multi-organ failure. A dose of 7 mg has caused death, but in other cases, people have recovered after consuming larger amounts.

Colchicum probably administered in food was used in 1855 by Catherine Wilson [10] to murder Maria Soames of London.

Atropine (Belladonna)

Belladonna (*Atropa belladonna*) is a plant whose Italian name translates as 'beautiful woman'. Indeed, drops extracted from the plant were used by women to dilate their eye pupils to make them appear more alluring. More ominously, *Atropa* in the plant's Latin name refers to Atropos, one of the three fates who cut the thread of life spun by her two sisters, and the plant's common name is deadly nightshade.

Belladonna liniment is applied externally to treat neuralgia (nerve pain). Drops were used to dilate the pupils allowing the interior of the eye to be examined. Belladonna was a constituent of cough mixtures for whooping cough and bronchitis, helping to control coughing and to dry up mucus.

Atropine is an alkaloid extracted from the plant. It has been used to counter the effects of poisoning by opium, and by muscarine, the poisonous component of some mushrooms. Atropine is absorbed by the gastro-intestinal tract and can also be administered intravenously. Partly oxidised in the liver, it is excreted in urine. Death has been reported after doses of less than 10 mg for children and smaller than 100 mg for adults.

A function of the parasympathetic nervous system is to inhibit heart action and encourage digestive action. Atropine, blocking the effect of the neurotransmitter acetylcholine, antagonises this system. As a result heart action is augmented and digestive action is encouraged. In very small doses atropine relieves spasm by paralysing the muscles of digestion, and raises heart rate. In general, it has an excitor effect followed by a depressant effect on the motor areas of the brain. Symptoms of atropine poisoning are in a sense extremes of the effects of tiny doses. Mouth and throat become very dry, pupils dilate, and heart rate increases. Excitement and delirium are accompanied by weakness. Later symptoms are cerebral depression, paralysis, coma and the gradual cessation of breathing and heartbeat. In treating atropine poisoning, barbiturates are used to help to control the excitement stage of the poisoning.

Swiss nurse Marie Jeanneret [13] was convicted in 1868 of the murder of her seven patients with belladonna, probably with sadistic motives, and imprisoned.

Aconite

Also known as wolf's bane or monk's hood, aconite (*Aconitum napelus*) grows in North America and Europe. Ancient Greeks are thought to have named the plant after the rocks (aconas) on which it grew. Aconite, or aconitine, is a poisonous alkaloid extracted from the plant in the form of a white crystalline powder.

In the past, tinctures of aconite were taken in the early onset of fevers, partly because they promote sweating. Applied to the skin as a liniment, aconite was used as a counter irritant to relieve rheumatic or similar pain. It appears that by stimulating nerve endings, aconite relieves pain in muscles served by the same nerve route, possibly by setting up pain impulses from the skin which alter the effect of the original pain from other sites. However, the danger of harm was high if the liniment was used liberally especially on broken skin.

If taken orally, aconite creates a sensation of warmth or tingling in the mouth, throat and stomach and skin. Later symptoms are feelings of coldness to the skin, giddiness, restlessness, vomiting and diarrhoea, convulsions, and increasing breathing problems as the muscles that control respiration become paralysed. Death ensues from about eight minutes to four hours after the poison is taken. A fatal dose of aconite can be as little as 1 mg, or about 5–10 ml of tincture. Stimulants such as atropine are sometimes given to try to counteract aconite poisoning.

For financial gain, morphine addict Dr. George Lamson [17] killed his brother-in-law with aconite in a Dundee cake while visiting him at his school in Wimbledon, England. Royal Navy surgeon Dr. Edward Pritchard [12] killed his mother-in-law and his wife with aconite (and antimony). Much more recently (in 2010) Lakvir Singh [93] was convicted of poisoning her lover Lakhvinder Cheema by lacing his curry with aconite probably brought back to London when she made a trip to India.

Strychnine

Obtained from plants of the genus *Strychnos*, strychnine is a vegetable alkaloid having an extremely bitter taste. In tiny doses, it acts as a nerve stimulant. It has been used medicinally as a tonic, or as a 'bitter' to improve appetite. Taken by mouth, strychnine is quickly absorbed by the intestine but only slowly excreted, partly unchanged in urine. Some of the substance is destroyed by the liver.

About 100 mg taken orally represents a fatal dose, the minimum lethal dose being about 36 mg.

Strychnine stimulates the central nervous system, and inhibits the nerves of the spinal cord from counteracting over stimulation. Consequently, overdoses cause twitching and then convulsions. The cortex is affected and senses are heightened. After central nervous system stimulation there is a period of depression. Following poisoning, convulsions seize the sufferer so that the body is arched back with arms and legs extended (opisthotonic convulsions). Facial muscles contract producing a characteristic sardonic grin. While this wave of convulsions is taking place, the senses are heightened. Contraction of the diaphragm and related muscles prevent breathing while spasms persist. Typically convulsions last for a minute or two with ten or fifteen minutes of respite. Death usually occurs after the second to the fifth seizure. Asphyxiation is brought about by the action of the poison on the respiratory muscles. A massive overdose of strychnine can kill suddenly without convulsions. In attempting to treat strychnine poisoning, injections of a rapidly acting barbiturate and muscle relaxants are given (Farrell 1993a).

Dr. William Palmer [8] of Rugeley, England poisoned his gambling companion John Cook, for which he was publicly hanged before a crowd of some 30,000 spectators in 1856. Glasgow born Dr. Neill Cream [22] practiced medicine in Chicago, where he murdered the husband of his mistress and was given a life prison sentence. On his release he moved to London, where he poisoned four prostitutes using strychnine for which he went to the scaffold in 1872. Farmer Walter Horsford [27] killed his cousin, a widow, Mrs. Holmes with strychnine sent to her through the post with instructions to take it. She was pregnant with his child and he was afraid that his wife would find out.

In County Armagh, Ireland, using strychnine, Sarah Anne Pearson and Agnes Black [30] murdered 74 year old Alice Pearson (who was Sarah's mother in law and Agnes's mother). Monetary gain was the motive. Jean Pierre Vaquier [45] a French guest at the Blue Anchor public house in Byfleet, Surrey, England, had recently become the lover of Mabel Jones the landlord's wife. He killed Mr. Jones by adding strychnine to the landlord's hangover cure. Vaquier was executed in 1924. In Lincolnshire, England, Gamekeeper's daughter Ethel Major [49] killed her lorry (truck) driver husband with strychnine and misled the attending physician by claiming that her husband's convulsions were symptoms of epilepsy, a condition which he had kept secret for fear of losing his job.

Opium and Morphine

Opium is an extract of the poppy (*Papaver somniferum*) Somnius being the Roman god of sleep. A milky juice is tapped from the unripe head of the plant and dries into a brownish elastic substance which is then scraped off and collected as raw opium. This contains many alkaloids, mainly morphine (about 10%) but also codeine, narcotine and others.

Opium was eaten or smoked as a soporific in China and elsewhere into the 1900s. Medical uses included Dover's powder to encourage sweating and induce sleep in less severe cases of fever. The principal active ingredient in opium is morphine and the two substances are essentially the same in relation to absorption, distribution, excretion, action, and symptoms.

French school teacher Eugène Chantrelle [16], having killed his English wife Elizabeth Dyer with opium was hanged in 1878.

Morphine or morphia is an alkaloid derived from opium. Until 1803, crude opium as used in medicine until Friederich Setürner isolated its principal active ingredient. Following tests first on animals and later on humans, Setürner noticed that one effect was cerebral depression. He called the substance morphine after Morpheus the Roman god of sleep and dreams.

Physicians administered morphine orally as a pain killer. Morphine acetate (morphine combined with acetic acid) was used as was morphine to relieve pain, to sedate, to ease diarrhoea, and to sooth coughing. But as morphine became popular, it was noted that some patients could become addicted to the drug. In 1848, the invention of the syringe allowed morphine to be injected directly into the bloodstream which was initially thought to reduce the risk of dependence but in fact did not. Problems of addiction were exacerbated by the free availability of morphine.

In the twentieth century, morphine became a substitute for opium. As well as being an easer of pain, it helped to control coughs and diarrhoea. It also induces euphoria in the dying and eases anxiety in conditions such as shock or heart failure. Morphine is absorbed by the alimentary tract when taken by mouth and absorbed more quickly when injected under the skin. Detoxicated in the liver, it is excreted in urine.

As a cerebral depressant, morphine dampens down aspects of the central nervous system so disrupting concentration and inducing lethargy and sleep. It depresses respiration and the cough reflex. At the same time, the drug stimulates other aspects of the central nervous system, causing eye pupils to contract, and inducing vomiting. This central respiratory depression can lead to coma and death. In treating morphine poisoning, drugs are used to try to prevent respiratory failure.

In 1823, French physician Dr. Edme Castaing [3] murdered Hippolyte Ballet for financial gain by adding morphine acetate powder to Ballet's wine and later a medicinal 'draught'. Becoming the first physician to be convicted of murder using morphine, Castaing was guillotined in 1823, aged only 27 years. New York based Scottish physician Dr. Robert Buchanan [25] killed his second wife Anna with morphine, inherited a fortune, and a month later re-married his first wife arousing suspicions which led to his conviction and eventual electrocution in Sing Sing Prison. In 1891, in New York, medical student Carlysle Harris [24] killed his wife by tampering with the constituents of drug capsules that she was taking, so they contained a lethal dose of morphine.

London chemist assistant Arthur Deveureux [31] killed his wife and twin sons with morphine and placed their bodies in a trunk which he deposited in a furniture repository before moving to a different part of the county. His mother-in-law's suspicions led to his arrest and conviction. Nursing home manager Dorothea Waddingham [50] killed two patients with morphine for monetary gain. In England over a period of decades, Dr. Harold Shipman [81] killed some 250 of his patients, often using overdoses of morphine based drugs, before being brought to trial and convicted in 1999.

Cyanide, Potassium Cyanide and Prussic Acid

Cyanides are poisonous salts of hydrocyanic acid (prussic acid). In nature, the seeds of apples, peaches, cherries and almonds and other fruits and nuts contain cyanide compounds. Cherry laurel (*Prunus laurocerasus*) was used by entomologists to prepare killing bottles for collecting insects. Entire, crushed, fresh leaves were enclosed on a corked bottle where they gave off hydrocyanic acid. Cherry laurel water produced through the water distillation of cherry laurel was used for treating coughs digestive problems, and insomnia. (There is at least one case of its use as a homicidal poison in the 1700s). If leaves of the wild black cherry tree (*Prunus serotina*) are chewed and swallowed, the amygdalin they contain is broken down by stomach enzymes and turns into lethal hydrogen cyanide.

One compound of cyanide is the salt potassium cyanide which is used to case-harden steel in electroplating, and to extract gold and silver from its ores. Another salt, sodium cyanide, is used in prison gas chambers where a pellet of the compound is dropped into a receptacle containing dilute sulphuric acid to produce hydrogen cyanide gas. While sodium and potassium salts of hydrogen cyanide are inert, water or gastric acid immediately hydrolyses them into hydrogen cyanide. As a consequence, if cyanide salts are swallowed, the hydrogen cyanide produced is both absorbed by the gastro-intestinal tract and inhaled into the air passages.

A minimum lethal dose is estimated to be between 0.7 and 3.5 mg per kilo of body weight. A dose of 50 mg (about the weight of a postage stamp) contains ten billion billion molecules (in US terms) or ten milliard milliard molecules (in UK measures where milliard equals one thousand million). This constitutes about ten cyanide molecules to every body cell.

Cyanide acts by inhibiting the bodily enzyme cytochrome oxidase and preventing the body from using oxygen, even though it is present in adequate amounts. Death may be caused by respiratory failure because lack of oxygen damages the nerve cells of the respiratory centre of the brain and because the muscle walls of the heart are affected. Exposure to hydrogen cyanide gas can bring about unconsciousness in about ten seconds and death in a minute owing to cardiac arrhythmias and ventricular asystole, which affect control of heart beat. Once cyanide is administered, symptoms appear in a few minutes: giddiness, limb weakness, and blue coloration of the lips and face being pronounced. Heart action slows and becomes irregular and after around three minutes, convulsions may occur before breathing and heartbeat cease. As an antidote to cyanide poisoning, nitrates may be used to convert the cyanide in the blood into a harmless substance, cyanmethaemoglobin.

In 1845, Quaker John Tawell [5] killed an unwanted mistress with prussic acid added to a bottle of 'stout'. Richard Brinkley [33] intended to kill a certain Reginald Parker with stout laced with prussic acid, but the beer was in fact drunk by Parker's visiting landlord and wife who both died.

In the US, Reverend Clarence Richeson [38] killed a girlfriend with potassium cyanide. Infantry officer Adolph Hofrichter [36] posted potassium cyanide capsules as a supposed aphrodisiac from a pharmacist, to officers whom he felt had been preferentially promoted above him. One of these Captain Richard Mader died as a result. In 1939, Michigan pastor Reverend Frank Sipple [54] killed his daughter Dorothy with a cyanide capsule and her death was put down to a heart attack. Her murder went undiscovered until 1946 when the pastor under police interrogation for a different offence, admitted killing Dorothy. In the years following 1941 during the German occupation of France, physician Dr. Marcel Petiot [55] pretended to be part of the French Resistance facilitating anyone wishing to leave the country. Unsuspecting victims would visit his surgery at night with their money and possessions. Under the pretext of vaccinating the victim against diseases prevalent in the country to which they were planning to flee, Petiot injected them with cyanide. The law caught up with Petiot in 1946 when he was guillotined for murdering twenty four people over several years.

In Japan, in 1948, Sadamichi Hirasawa [56], posing as an official, killed bank staff with cyanide laced liquid which he convinced them were needed to help control an outbreak of dysentery, and then he robbed the place. On Halloween 1974, in Texas, Ronald Clark O'Bryan [73] poisoned his eight year old son with potassium cyanide laced candy in order to claim life insurance. In 1986, in Washington, Stella Nickell [75] poisoned her husband Bruce with cyanide to gain financially from his life insurance, his death being put down to emphysema. As accidental death paid more than death from natural causes, Stella who had reported that her husband had died after having taken Excedrin™ capsules, then tampered with similar capsules in local stores as a result of which Susan Snow, a local bank manager died after taking such capsules. Eventually, Stella Nickel was charged with product tampering and sentenced to two 90 year prison sentences. Cyanide poisoning was one of the murder methods used by serial killer Donald Harvey [76] who also poisoned with arsenic, insulin, and morphine and used suffocation and other methods. Although he pleaded guilty to 24 killings, official estimates are that he killed even more victims, mainly patients at hospitals in Kentucky and Cincinnati between 1970 and 1987. Sentenced to serve 28 life sentences, he was imprisoned in Toledo, Ohio. Ryan Furlough [86] an eighteen year old Maryland high school student, who was in love with the girlfriend of his friend Benjamin Vassilev, poisoned his rival with cyanide laced soft drink. In India, K.D. Kempanna [94] also known as Mallika and by several other aliases used cyanide to poison six women temple worshipers between 1997 and 2007. Posing as a pious devotee familiar with temple rituals, she befriended the wealthy women and frequented temples with them. Then suggesting a visit to an out of the way temple, she would on arrival there add cyanide to their food and rob them of their valuables. Dr. Robert Ferrante [97] poisoned his wife Autumn Klein with cyanide for which he was sentenced in 2015. Jessica Wongso [100] gave her friend Wayan Salihin cyanide in her coffee at a café in Jakarta, Indonesia, out of jealousy over friend's success and new husband.

Digitalis

Foxglove (*Digitalis purpurea*) is an attractive plant whose Latin name indicates its noticeable features: it has purple colouring and it is finger shaped (the word 'digit' is of course still used to mean finger). Digitalis the poison is extracted from its leaves. As early as the 1700 s it was known to be used in a herb tea to treat 'dropsy' a condition in which excessive amounts of fluid accumulate under the skin, exerting its effect by causing large quantities of urine to be passed. It was only in more recent times that digitalis came to be used to treat heart failure, and other conditions characterised by rapid and irregular heartbeat.

The drugs digitoxin and digoxin are extracts of digitalis which have a more powerful effect than simpler plant preparations. A lethal dose of digitoxin is 3–5 mg, that of digoxin is 5–25 mg and that of most digitalis preparations is much greater (about 2.5 gm).

Digitalis increases activity of muscular tissue particularly the heart and arterioles (small blood vessels). In therapeutic doses, it strengthens each heartbeat and lengthens, 'rest' beats. Increased blood flow leads to the kidneys producing more urine, so decreasing 'dropsy' where this is the result of heart problems. Toxic amounts cause nausea, vomiting and blurred vision. Heartbeat becomes irregular, breathing is laboured, and the individual may become convulsed or unconscious before death ensues.

A case of homicidal poisoning using digitalis was that of Frenchman Dr. Edmund de la Pommerais [11] who was guillotined in 1864 for the murder of his mistress Seraphine de Pawr.

Nicotine

An alkaloid derived from the tobacco plant (*Nicotiana tabacum*), nicotine is named after Jean Nicot who introduced tobacco to the French Court. An oily liquid, it is pale yellow to clear in colour. In the past it was widely used as an insecticide.

Nicotine is readily absorbed through the gastro-intestinal tract when swallowed. If injected subcutaneously or if it passes through the surface of the skin, its absorption is slower. It is excreted in urine and sweat. A fatal dose for an adult is between 40 and 60 mg. With acute poisoning, death can ensue within minutes. Nicotine first stimulates then paralyses the autonomic ganglia (clusters of nerve cells in the autonomic nervous system regulating involuntary action and some internal organs).

It also affects the central nervous system, small doses encouraging respiration, but large doses causing convulsions and arresting the muscles used for respiration. Heart failure and death are the consequences. Symptoms of nicotine poisoning, reflecting its action, include vomiting, convulsions, paralysis and eventually death.

Count Hippolyte de Bocarme [6], a Belgian nobleman, killed his brother-in-law Gustave Fougnies for financial gain using nicotine for which he went to the guillotine in 1851. Paul Marshall Curry [95], a nuclear power plant engineer in the US, gave small doses of nicotine to his wife Linda over an extended period then administered a lethal injection of the poison. While the crime took place in 1995, conviction had to await fresh evidence, sentence being passed in 2014.

Hyoscine

Hyoscine is an alkaloid derived from henbane (*Hyoscyamus niger*) a plant occasionally found for example, on waste ground in southern England. Therapeutically, hyoscine was used to calm sickness (such as sea sickness). Taken with morphine, hyoscine was used to discourage mania, and was in the 1920s sometimes used to induce a twilight sleep during child delivery. Administered by hypodermic needle in the form of hydrobromide it was used as a sedative. Hyoscine hydrobromide has an anti-aphrodisiac effect. Hyoscine is an anticholine, blocking the effect of the nerve –muscle transmitting substance acetylcholine, and depressing the central nervous system. A lethal dose of hyoscine hydrobromide is between a quarter and a half a grain.

In one of the most famous of all poison cases, Michigan born Dr. Hawley Harvey Crippen [35] was hanged in London in 1910 for killing his wife Cora Turner with hyoscine before eloping with his lover Ethel Le Neve. Over a hundred years later, DNA investigation of a specimen used at the trial raised questions about the remains found at Crippen's home (Foran, Wills, Kiley, Jackson and Trestrail III, 2011).

Animal Poisons (Zootoxins)

Poisoning from animals generally occurs as it were, in nature as when an individual is stung or bitten by a venomous snake, insect, spider or fish. White et. al (2008) discuss these poisons as well as antivenoms. But the use of animal poisons in homicides seems to be unusual and the examples discussed below involve not 'natural' venoms but the use of a powder made from a beetle *Cantharis vesicatoria*, and of the pancreatic hormone insulin.

Cantharides

Cantharides is a powder made from the dried body and wings of a beetle, *Cantharis vesicatoria*, found in Spain, Italy and the south of Russia. The creature's Spanish habitat gave the powder its common name of 'Spanish fly'. In the East, the dried Chinese or Indian blistering beetle (*Mylabris sidea*) is a source of cantharides. In both sources, the active component is cantharadin.

As an irritant, cantharides acts on the parts of the body with which it comes into contact. When passing out of the system, it irritates the urinary and genital organs, and for this reason was erroneously thought to be an aphrodisiac. Its medical use was as a blistering agent applied to the skin as a plaster or painted on as a blistering fluid. This was intended to ease severe pain such as that from sciatica or to encourage the absorption of fluid from thickened joints. It has also been used to remove warts and to treat verruca. Cantharidin solution was sometimes used in hair lotions to stimulate the scalp.

Fatality has been caused by as little as one and a half to three grains but in other cases people have recovered after much larger doses. Taken orally, cantharides causes burning pain in the throat and stomach and difficulty in swallowing. Nausea, vomiting, colic, bloody diarrhoea, and blood in the urine are further symptoms before collapse and death.

In London, in 1954, Arthur Ford [60] the office manager of a manufacturing chemist made a tragic mistake of thinking that cantharides was an aphrodisiac. Surreptitiously giving cantharides laced sweets/candies to a secretary to whom he was attracted he killed her (and another secretary who also took a doctored sweet). Convicted of manslaughter rather than murder, it was judged that he had no intention to kill.

Insulin

In the human body, insulin is a hormone produced by the pancreas, helping keep blood sugar at normal levels. With increased blood glucose the so called Beta cells in the pancreas are signalled to secrete insulin. The insulin attaches to cells and signals them to absorb blood sugar to be used for energy. Insulin was isolated by Nicholai Paulsen in Romania in 1920 and by Banting and Best in Canada in 1923, since when various sources have been used. Increasingly, human insulin is made available through genetic engineering. Diabetes mellitus is a condition in which blood sugar levels are too high, associated with having insufficient insulin produced in the body. When insulin is depleted, blood glucose concentration increases and glucose is passed out in the urine. Injections of insulin enable the blood sugar to be used fully. Where too much insulin is taken, then blood sugar levels can be reduced too much (hypoglycaemia). Because glucose is an important source of energy for the brain, a deficiency can damage the central nervous system, leading to convulsions, coma, and death. An overdose can be treated by dextrose or ordinary sugar to restore the balance (Kumar and Clarke 2016).

In England in 1957, Kenneth Barlow [63] injected his wife with insulin (perhaps persuading her it was ergometrine an abortifacient) rendering her unconscious before drowning her in her bath. In Stockport, England, in 2015, a nurse Victorino

Chua [98] was found guilty of murdering two patients with overdoses of insulin at his hospital. Further insulin cases are described by Marks and Richmond (2007).

Bacterial Poisons

Bacteria and Bacterial Poisons

The term bacteria may be understood broadly to include micro-organisms in the form of microscopic forms of plant life, as well as bacteria proper which are simple, primitive forms of micro-organism. Micro-organisms may be moulds, yeasts, bacteria, *Rickettsia*, and viruses. Moulds include microscopic fungi such as ring-worm which can grow in body tissue. Yeast of a particular type procures alcohol. Bacteria proper include organisms of different shapes – round, curved or rod-like. *Rickettsia* are organisms which cause disease and are larger than bacteria and *Rickettsia prowazekii* is the infecting agent of typhus. Viruses are minute agents causing diseases such as poliomyelitis and influenza.

Bacteria cause disease by producing toxins which are harmful to tissues. One group, endotoxins are retained in the bacterial cells and the bacteria can do damage wherever they are sited in the body, while another group, exotoxins (such as diphtheria) pass from the bacteria and are circulated throughout the body. Tuberculosis is caused by one of two micro bacteria: the human type which usually causes tuberculosis of the lungs, and the bovine type which causes abdominal tuberculosis. Typhoid fever and related diseases are brought about by *Salmonella typhi*, and similar organisms. Diphtheria is caused by *Corynebacterium diphtheria* which produces severe throat inflammation and other symptoms. Influenza is caused by virus.

Typhoid, Tuberculosis, and Diphtheria

Bacteria cause disease by producing toxins which are harmful to bodily tissues. Enteric fever is an acute illness associated with fever, abdominal discomfort and headache. Typhoid a typical form of enteric fever is brought about by *Salmonella typhi* transmitted in contaminated water or food. Symptoms of typhoid may include a high temperature, headache, stomach pain, aching muscles, feeling sick, poor appetite, either constipation or diarrhoea, confusion, and exhaustion. In developing countries, for up to 30% of people contracting enteric fever it can prove fatal.

Tuberculosis is caused by *Mycobacterium tuberculosis* and sometimes by *Mycobacterium bovis* or *Mycobacterium africanum*. This bacterium is able to invade cells and can be grown in a laboratory that is it is a facultative intracellular organism. It mainly affects the lungs but can act on other parts of the body too.

Symptoms may include a persistent cough producing blood, fever, fatigue and loss of appetite (Kumar and Clark 2016, pp. 86–87).

Diphtheria is caused by *Corynebacterium diphtheriae*. Symptoms may include severe throat inflammation, a thick grey membrane covering the throat, swollen neck glands (Lymph nodes), nasal discharge, and difficulty breathing or rapid breathing (See also Barlow et al. 2016, Chap. 11).

In France, Henry Girrard [42] an insurance dealer poisoned an insurance broker friend by injecting him with typhoid bacteria under the pretext of administering a tonic. American dentist and bacteriologist, Arthur Waite [40] dispatched his mother in law using diphtheria and tuberculosis bacteria (and killed his father-in-law with arsenic) for which he was electrocuted in 1917.

Drugs

Fentanyl

A synthetic opiate drug used as a tranquiliser and painkiller, fentanyl could also be considered with opium and morphine. Fentanyl is a powerful drug, 50–100 times stronger than morphine. It acts quickly and its effects are relatively short in duration. Used medicinally as a palliative it can be absorbed from a skin patch, as dissolving tablets, and as a mouth spray. In carefully monitored highly diluted doses it is used as an anaesthetic. Where it is used as a 'recreational' drug, it has led to overdoses and deaths. Indeed medical examiners determined that the musician Prince died from an accidental overdose in 2016. In veterinary practice fentanyl is used for example as an analgesic following an operation on a small animal such as a dog or cat. Symptoms of overdose include confusion and dizziness, vomiting, slowed heart rate and low blood pressure, respiratory arrest, coma and ultimately death (Centre for Disease Control and Prevention 2016).

Toxicologist Kristin Rossum [82] used fentanyl to poison her husband Greg de Villiers. It appears that she was concerned that he would reveal an affair she was having with the head toxicologist Michael Robertson, and her growing addiction to metaphine stolen from the coroner's laboratory. She was sentenced in 2002.

Methylphenobarbitone

A barbiturate, methylphenobarbitone is a white crystalline powder. Although tasteless and odourless, the drug is practically insoluble in water. Taken in tablet form, it is an anti-convulsant prescribed for epilepsy and has also been used to treat chronic alcoholism. In toxic doses, methylphenobarbitone causes respiratory depression, weakened heartbeat, loss of body heat, and coma. Death is brought about by paralysis of the respiratory centre of the brainstem.

In London, in 1953, Teresa Conroy [57] killed her epileptic son with carbon-monoxide gas (coal gas) and methylphenobarbitone (which he was taking as an epilepsy medication). Found guilty but insane, she was detained for an indefinite period.

Seconal Sodium

A white, odourless but bitter tasting powder, Seconal sodium is another name for the barbiturate quinalbarbitone. Barbituric acid yields several effective derivatives having a hypnotic effect, one of which, barbitone, began to be used in clinical practice in the early 1900s. Seconal sodium itself is used as a sedative taken orally in capsules of methyl cellulose. Absorbed by the gastro-intestinal tract, Seconal sodium is excreted in urine after the body has absorbed most of it (and in the normal course of events destroyed it). As with other barbiturates, Seconal sodium depresses the central nervous system. Acting on the higher centres first, it then works down the CNS mainly affecting the cerebral cortex and the thalamic region of the brain. Overdoses of Seconal sodium block autonomic nerves which regulate the functions of certain internal organs. An overdose also acts directly to depress the vascular smooth muscles.

Symptoms of Seconal sodium poisoning are failure of the circulatory system affecting the kidneys. Little or no urine is passed. The respiratory system fails and coma and death follow. Owing to central depression of respiratory centres in the brain stem, respiratory failure is almost invariably the cause of death where a fatal overdose is taken.

In England, John Armstrong [62] killed his baby son Terence with Seconal sodium in 1955 for which he was sentenced a year later.

Succinylcholine Chloride

Succinylcholine chloride (curacit) also known as suxamethonium chloride (sometimes abbreviated colloquially to 'sux') is a synthetic drug used to relax muscles. An off-white crystalline powder, it has little odour, a salty taste, and is soluble in water. Succinylcholine chloride is used intravenously in anaesthetics, being particularly useful in brief operations such as when a tube needs to be passed down the trachea to aid breathing.

A neuromuscular blocking agent, the drug paralyses the muscles for a brief period when administered in a small dose. It acts by depolarisation, preventing 'communication' between muscle and nerves. Overdose can cause irregular action of the heart: slow beats, extra contracting as opposed to resting phases, and even heart failure. This appears to relate to extra stimulation of the vagal nerve supplying branches to the heart and other organs. In treating succinylcholine chloride poisoning, blood transfusion may help to replace the nerve transmitting agent cholinesterase which is rendered inactive by the drug.

In 1967, a San Francisco court found anaesthetist Dr. Carl Coppolino [66] guilty of the second degree murder of his wife Carmela, through injecting her with succinylcholine chloride. Norwegian nursing home manager Arnfinn Nessett [72] was found guilty in 1982 of twenty one charges of poisoning residents of his nursing home with succinylcholine chloride. In the US, paediatric nurse Genene Jones [74] used succinylcholine to kill 15 month old Chelsea McClellan and heparin (a blood thinning drug) to murder another child Rolando Santos, and was suspected of many more deaths. Critical care nurse Charles Higgs [90] was, in 2006, found guilty of poisoning his wife former State Controller Kathy Augustine with succinylcholine chloride.

Vecuronium Bromide

Vecuronium bromide is a neuromuscular blocking agent acting as a muscle paralysing drug. It is used for similar purposes as succinylcholine chloride (curacit) being in the curariform class of drugs. Supplied in ampules of powder, it is dissolved and administered in solution by intravenous injection as part of anaesthesia. It is excreted in urine and in faeces. Overdose is highly dangerous. It is used non-medically as part of the mixture of poisons in a lethal injection for judicial execution in some US states.

Vecuronium bromide was used by Daisuke Mori [85] a nurse in Japan, who was sentenced to life imprisonment in 2004 for poisoning Yukiko Shimoyama an 89-year-old woman patient at the clinic in Izumi-ku, Sendai, where Mori worked. The nurse was also suspected of four attempted murders of patients in 2000.

Conclusion

The chapter considered plant poisons: colchicum seeds, atropine (belladonna), aconite, strychnine, opium and morphine, cyanide (and potassium cyanide and prussic acid), digitalis, nicotine and hyoscine. We looked at the animal poisons: cantharides, and insulin. Bacterial poisons: typhoid, tuberculosis and, diphtheria were discussed. Drugs considered were: fentanyl, methylphenobarbitone, Seconal, succinylcholine chloride, and vecuronium bromide. In all cases we referenced homicidal poisoners who have used these substances.

Suggested Activities

Review examples of cases from the glossary where the perpetrator used: plant poison, animal poison, and bacteria.

Key Texts

Kumar and Clark (2016) (9th edition) *Clinical Medicine* Philadelphia, PA, Elsevier Saunders

Most standard texts on clinical medicine have chapters covering infectious diseases. In such a chapter, this well illustrated book discusses typhus, tuberculosis and diphtheria and other conditions.

Nelson et al. (2007) (2nd. Edition) *Handbook of Poisonous and Injurious Plants* New York, Springer

Two of the authors are physicians and the third is a botanist. Their concise book includes references to aconite, belladonna, colchicum, digitalis, cyanogenic compound genera, henbane (hyoscine), nicotiana tabacum, and other plant poisons. Toxic mechanisms and poisons and poisoning syndromes are discussed.

United States Pharmacopeial Convention (2015) *United States Pharmacopeia* [*US Pharmacopeia National Formulary*]. Rockville, MD, United States Pharmacopeial Convention

Many countries have their pharmacopeia or national formulary. The US version is published annually and provides details of drugs including the ones discussed in the present chapter.

References

Barlow, G., Irving, W. L. & Moss, P. J. (2016). Infectious Disease. In P. Kumar & M. Clark (eds.), *Clinical medicine* (9th ed.) Philadelphia, PA: Elsevier Saunders.

Center for Disease Control and Prevention (2016). *Fentanyl.* Atlanta, Ga: CDCP.

Farrell, M. (1993a). What's your poison? *Solicitors' Journal*, p. 254.

Foran, D. R., Wills, B. E., Kiley, B. M., Jackson, C. B., & Trestrail, J. H., III. (2011). The conviction of Dr. Crippen: New forensic findings in a century old murder' (Case Report Criminalistics). *Journal of Forensic Sciences, 56*(1), 233–240.

Kumar, P., & Clark, M. (Eds.) (2016) *Clinical medicine* (9th ed.). Philadelphia, PA: Elsevier Saunders.

Marks, V., & Richmond, C. (2007) *Insulin murders: True life cases*. London: Royal Society of Medicine Press.

Nelson, L.S., Richard, D.S., & Balick, M.J. (2007). *Handbook of poisonous and injurious plants* (2nd ed.). New York, Springer.

United States Pharmacopeial Convention (2015). *United States Pharmacopeia [US Pharmacopeia National Formulary]*. Rockville, MD, United States: Pharmacopeial Convention.

White, J., Meier, J., & Warrell, D. A. (eds.) (2008). *Handbook of clinical toxicology of animal venoms and poisons* (2nd ed.). New York and London: CRC Press.

Chapter 6
Elements and 'Other Poisons'

Introduction

Some substances considered here are, for example arsenic and chloroform, while associated with poisons long in the past, are not only historical footnotes. Arsenic was used to kill a church worshiper in Portland, Maine in 2003. In England, two brothers murdered the lover of one of them with chloroform as recently as 2015.

Elements, Their Compounds and Derivatives

Arsenic

Arsenic and Its Properties

Elemental arsenic is a semimetal which although it can be found in its natural state separately is often combined with antimony and silver. It is normally recovered when other metals such as lead, copper and gold are smelted. Being inert, elemental arsenic is not toxic when swallowed because it is not absorbed into the system. Compounds of arsenic are quite a different matter. In fact arsenic compounds were known long before the element was isolated. Ancient Greeks, Romans and Arabs, used such compounds medicinally and as poisons. Arsenic compounds may be organic or inorganic.

Inorganic arsenicals are either trivalent (having three electrons available for bonding with other substances) or pentavalent (with five electrons for bonding). Among trivalent arsenicals, arsenic trioxide (white arsenic) is probably the best known. Sugar like in appearance, it is almost tasteless and when in the past it was readily available was a common choice for homicidal poisoning. White arsenic was

M. Farrell, *Criminology of Homicidal Poisoning*,
DOI 10.1007/978-3-319-59117-9_6

used as a rodent poison, and in insecticides and herbicides, and in the textile, glass and enamel industries. Another trivalent arsenical, cupric arsenate (Scheele's Green), is used in the manufacture of dyes and paints. Regarding pentavalent forms, potassium arsenate is a constituent of sheep dip and insect poison. Soil may be sterilised with lead arsenate, which is also used in paint (Farrell 1989).

Organic arsenicals were so called owing to the erroneous supposition that organic materials contained some vital force that inorganic ones lacked. When this notion was discredited in the early 1800s, the distinction faded in importance and by the end of the nineteenth century an 'organic substance' simply meant a carbon compound. Cacodylate, the first known organic arsenical was identified in 1842. The pioneering work of German physician and scientist Paul Ehrlich (1854–1915) including his discovery of Arsphenamine (606) laid the foundations for chemotherapy. Organic arsenicals were found to be less toxic that inorganic forms and more easily absorbed into the body, but still damaged certain bodily cells. It was discovered that certain toxic substances could be 'attracted' to sites of infection or disease where they could work without major harm to bodily functions. Around 1911, Ehrlich discovered Salvarsal an arsenic compound that became the first cure for syphilis.

Some arsenicals such as arsenic trioxide dissolve only slowly in water. Consequently, when they enter the body the speed at which they are absorbed depends on how finely they are powdered. If the powder is coarse, it tends to be less toxic because it can be excreted in faeces before it has the chance to dissolve. In contrast, arsenates such as potassium arsenate are more water soluble and therefore better absorbed.

Bodily distribution of arsenic is affected by the particular arsenical administered and the period over which doses have been taken. Arsenic is predominantly stored in heart, lung, liver and kidney tissue. A high concentration is also found in hair, nails, bones and teeth. This is because keratin, a natural substance found in these body parts, contains a high proportion of sulphur atoms to which arsenic particularly binds. Within only a few hours of being administered, arsenic begins to be laid down in the hair, where signs of it can remain for years. Arsenic is excreted mainly in urine.

Regarding the action of arsenic, trivalent arsenicals primarily binds to sulphur atoms in the body's enzymes. They inhibit suphydril containing enzyme systems essential to normal cellular metabolism. Pentavalent arsenicals compete in the cells for inorganic phosphate. Substituting themselves for phosphate, they combine with an organic compound to form a derivative that is quickly broken down (arseniolysis).

Where arsenic poisoning is *acute*, the early signs can include burning lips, tightening of the throat and difficulty in swallowing. Severe gastric pains, violent vomiting and excessive watery diarrhoea follow. Kidneys become inflamed, and proteins and blood appear in the urine which is passed only sparingly. Raging thirst and muscular craps ensue. As fluid is lost through vomiting and diarrhoea, symptoms of 'shock' appear. Coma and death follow. Where poisoning is very severe, death can occur in an hour but more commonly severe poisoning kills in around 24 h.

With *chronic* arsenic poisoning, an abnormal quantity of fluid accumulates beneath the skin especially the eyelids and face. (In the past, this was mistaken for healthy weight gain leading to arsenic being taken as a tonic). Other signs are loss of appetite, nausea, vomiting and diarrhoea. The membrane covering the front of the eye (conjunctiva) and the mucus membranes of the nose become inflamed and itchy, and the mouth becomes sore. Later symptoms include anaemia and cirrhosis of the liver. Jaundice becomes evident as bile pigment deposited in the deep layers of the skin turns its surface yellow. (Bile, a fluid made in the liver and stored in the gallbladder, aids digestion by breaking down fats to be digestible). Peripheral neuritis, a form of nerve inflammation, develops. Numbness and tingling occurs in the limbs, especially in the feet, sometimes causing a high stepping gait.

The minimal recorded lethal dose of arsenic is about 200 mg an amount that can be held on the tip on a knife blade. As a medical procedure, chelation therapy is used to remove heavy metals from the body. For arsenic, dimercapto-propane sulphonate (DMPS) or dimercaptosuccinic acid (DMSA) may be used.

Arsenic Poisoners in North America

Arsenic has been used by many poisoners over the centuries (Farrell 1990). In the US in 1898, Cordelia Botkin [28] sent arsenic impregnated chocolates by post to her lover's wife, Mary Dunning, killing her and, inadvertently, Mary's sister with whom Mary shared the confections. Johan Hoch [32] the 'Stockyards Bluebeard' was convicted in Chicago of the arsenic poisoning of his wife, Julia Walcker-Hoch. Mary Creighton and Everett Applegate [52] poisoned Everett's wife Ada with arsenic.

In Hartford, Connecticut, nursing home manager Amy Archer-Gilligan [41] was found guilty of the arsenic poisoning of Michael Gilligan (her second husband), and four residents of the home. Nannie Doss [61] of Oklahoma killed 11 people with arsenic: her mother, two sisters, two children, a nephew and five husbands and was apprehended when she had murdered her fifth husband after the attending physician became suspicious. When in 1979 secretary Marie Hilley [70] tried killing her daughter with arsenic injections, police investigations revealed that in 1975 she had poisoned her husband with the substance for life insurance money. After skipping bail, fabricating her own death and evading justice, she was finally convicted.

North Carolina police investigating the illness of Reverend Dwight Moore, the second husband of Blanche Moore [78] found that he was suffering arsenic poisoning. When the bodies of her boyfriend Raymond Reid and her first husband were exhumed it emerged that both died of arsenic poisoning years earlier. Convicted of murdering her boyfriend, Blanche was sentenced to death and in 2015 was still on death row.

Arrested in 1997, American physician Dr. Michael Swango [80] was found guilty of four murders and sentenced to life imprisonment. It is suspected that he carried out other killings of patients and colleagues between 1981 and 1997 using arsenic and various drugs. In 2000, Ann Miller Kontz [89] a research chemist in North Carolina poisoned her husband Eric Miller, a paediatric AIDS researcher, with arsenic in order to be with her lover. In 2003 in Portland, Maine following internal disputes at the Lutheran Church, farmer Daniel Bondeson [83] killed Walter Morrill aged 78 a fellow church worshiper, with arsenic administered in the after service coffee. Fifteen other church members also became ill. Bondeson shot himself leaving a suicide note confessing the crime a few days after the killing claiming that he just wanted to make others ill.

In Canada, Dr. William King [9], having fallen in love with one of his women patients, killed his wife with arsenic.

Arsenic Poisoners in England and Ireland

In England one-time nurse Mary Cotton [14] may have committed several murders motivated variously by monetary gain or the desire to replace one spouse or lover with another. Found guilty of poisoning her stepson with arsenic, she was hanged. After 9 years, the marriage of American Florence Maybrick [21] and her much older English cotton broker husband James was running into difficulties. In 1889, James died at the couple's home in Liverpool, England of arsenic poisoning. Controversially found guilty of his murder, Florence's death sentence was commuted to penal servitude for life.

Insurance agent Frederick Seddon [87] poisoned his lodger Eliza Barrow with arsenic for financial gain. She had made substantial amounts of money over to him in exchange for a life time annuity which of course would not have to be paid after her death. Major Herbert Armstrong [43] a solicitor in a Welsh border town murdered his wife Katherine with arsenic. Cornish insurance salesman Edward Black [44] poisoned his wife and fled their home three days before she died but was later apprehended. Charlotte Bryant [51] was hanged in 1936 for poisoning her farm labourer husband Frederick probably with arsenical weed killer. At a US air base in Norfolk, England, Air Force Master Sergeant Marcus Marymont [65] poisoned his wife with arsenic when she discovered that he was having an affair with another woman. Found guilty at a court martial, Marymont was returned home to serve a life prison sentence in Kansas.

In Ireland, in 1887, 62-year-old Dr. Philip Cross [20] poisoned his wife with arsenic in order to marry Mary Skinner the 20-year-old former governess to his six children.

Arsenic Poisoners in France, Germany and Elsewhere

In France, in 1840, Marie Lafarge [4] killed her husband with arsenic and was sentenced to life imprisonment. French housemaid Hélèna Jégado [7] poisoned a fellow servant girl Rosalie Sarrazin with arsenic from jealousy and was accused of two previous murders. German housekeeper Anna Zwanziger [2] was publicly decapitated by sword after being found guilty the arsenic poisoning of Frau Glaser a judge's wife, another employer Judge Grohmann, and Frau Gebhardt a magistrate's wife.

English ex-patriate Edith Carew [26] living in Japan in 1896 poisoned her husband and was sentenced to penal servitude for life. In 1911 in colonial India, Dr. Henry Clark and his lover Augusta Fullam [39] poisoned Augusta's husband with arsenic and a year later had Clarke's wife assassinated with a sword. South African Maria Groesbeek [67] poisoned her first husband Christian Burys with 'Antexit' arsenical ant poison so that she could marry the younger Gerhard Groesbeek. In 1932, South African nurse Daisy de Melker [46] poisoned her son William Cowle with arsenic in a flask of coffee.

Antimony and Tartar Emetic

A brittle, bluish white semimetal, antimony has a flaky, crystalline texture. Organic antimony compounds may be trivalent (having three electrons available for bonding) or pentavalent (with five electrons available for bonding). Trivalent antimony compounds include antimony potassium tartrate (tartar emetic) which comprises colourless crystals or white powder which is sweet tasting but odourless. Pentavalent antimony compounds include sodium antimony gluconate.

Cosmetic and medicinal uses of antimony have been known for millennia. Right up to the twentieth century, tartar emetic and other salts of antimony were used as powerful emetics. Previously used in cough medicines, antimony is now considered too toxic for this purpose. Trivalent organic antimony was used to treat the tropical disease bilharzia, and pentavalent organic antimony was a treatment for leishmaiasis, a group of tropical diseases. Antimony is used in paint, enamel and lacquer and in the glass and rubber industries.

Absorbed slowly from the gastrointestinal tract, antimony is distributed to give high concentrations in the liver and thyroid. It is excreted mainly in urine. Trivalent antimony compounds are more toxic than pentavalent ones and death has occurred following an intravenous injection of only 2 grains of tartar emetic. Trivalent antimony links itself to sulphydril groups of atoms in bodily cells to form the so-called thioantimonates and binds itself to red blood cells. This breaks down key elements of cell structure.

Very small doses of antimony act as an expectorant, clearing secretions from air passages by stimulating the salivary and bronchial glands, but also causing nausea. Acute and chronic antimony poisoning produces symptoms similar to those of arsenic and lead. Antimony which is still in the stomach can be made into a precipitate by calcium hydroxide or magnesium oxide.

Tartar emetic (Potassium antimony tartrate) is a salt of antimony which in tiny doses was used as its name suggests as an emetic. Its absorption, distribution, excretion and toxicity are similar to that of antimony. Symptoms of poisoning with emetic tartar are similar to those for lead or arsenic. The action of the poison includes an irritant effect on the mucus membranes of the stomach, inducing vomiting.

In England, George Chapman (Severin Klosowski) [29] a publican, murdered his barmaid lover Maud Marsh with antimony for which he was hanged.

Copper and Copper Sulphate

Copper has been prized as a metal since ancient times and modern uses exploit its attractive sheen as an ornamental material, and its conductivity to heat and electricity. Being an 'essential' element, copper exists in all organisms. It is necessary for blood formation, is contained in several enzymes and is present in all bodily tissue especially brain, heart, liver, kidney and hair.

Salts of copper such as copper sulphate have been employed since the days of ancient Egypt where they were used to treat conjunctivitis. Once used as emetics, salts of copper continue to be utilised as pigments in manufacturing ceramics and textiles, and as fungicides, germicides and insecticides.

Taken by mouth, copper sulphate is absorbed by the gastrointestinal tract. It is not one of the most toxic poisons, a relatively large 10 g being a possible lethal dose. Symptoms of copper sulphate poisoning include cramps, convulsions, coma and eventually death. One treatment for such poisoning is potassium ferrocyanide which combines with the copper to produce copper ferrocyanide which is insoluble. Other treatments are white of egg, milk, tartaric acid or magnesia.

Parisian pharmacist Pierre Moreau [15] poisoned his wife with copper sulphate to inherit her money and was guillotined in 1874.

Phosphorus and Organic Phosphorus Compound

Phosphorus

A white, waxy non-metallic element, phosphorus turns yellow when exposed to light. At normal temperatures, it combusts slowly, becoming luminous. Indeed the Greek words 'phos' means 'light' and 'phorus' conveys 'bringing' while the derived Latin 'phosphorus' refers to the 'morning star'.

Red phosphorus used in safety matches is fairly benign.

Yellow (white) phosphorus however is fatal in a dose as low as 50 mg. In England, Victorian match girls suffered phosphorus necrosis (gangrene of the lower jawbone) because of the phosphorus fumes associated with their trade. With this 'phossy jaw', pieces of bone were known to crumble away. Phosphorus has been used in industrial chemical processes and in rat poison.

Yellow phosphorus tastes unpleasant and has a sulphurous odour but has been administered as a poison in spirits and strong coffee which sufficiently disguise it. Although only a little soluble in water, the substance is more soluble in alcohol or in organic fluids such as olive oil. Taken by mouth, phosphorus is absorbed by the intestinal tract and distributed to internal organs where it particularly damages the liver. Its initial action is as an irritant while later as an essentially protoplasmic poison it breaks up cells in the liver and other internal organs. Acute poisoning indications include a garlic smell to the breath, vomit and faeces which may be luminescent, burning pains to the stomach, convulsions and coma. After one or two days, the symptoms may seem to subside before the delayed effects of the poison assert themselves as jaundice, collapse, coma and eventually death. As a treatment for phosphorus poisoning, copper sulphate has been used.

In England, in 1953, Louisa Merrifield [58] used rat poison containing phosphorus to murder the elderly Sarah Anne Ricketts, to whom she and her husband were housekeepers. Mary Wilson [64] was convicted of murdering Oliver Leonard (her second husband) and Ernest Wilson (her third husband) with elemental phosphorus in rat and beetle poison.

Organic Phosphorus Compound E605 and Dichlorvos

Chemist Gerhard Schroeder, at the Bayer works in Leverkusen, Germany, developed organic phosphorus compounds E605, which were used as insecticides. Following World War II, American troops seized stocks and the insecticides were developed in the US. The compound E605 goes under many names. Its chemical label is diethyl p-nitrophenyl phosphorothionate, while its common name is Parathion. Other alternative names include: DNTP, Etilon, Niran, Folidol, Thiophos 3422, Paraphos and SNP. By the 1950s, the substance was being used extensively in Florida citrus plantations and sold worldwide. In 1948 when the poison was marketed back to Germany, it was under its old name of E605. Its action is as an acetylcholinesterase inhibitor which inhibits the acetylcholinesterase enzyme from breaking down acetylcholine, so increasing the action of the neurotransmitter acetylcholine (and its duration).

German chemists devised tests detecting E605 in the early 1950s. For example to show its presence in blood, the substance was treated with caustic soda, turning yellow if the test was positive. Symptoms of E605 poisoning are similar to those for hydrogen cyanide: convulsions, and paralysis of the respiratory centres. Other symptoms include constriction of the eye pupils, slowed heartbeat and excessive salivation.

German chemical factory worker Christa Lehman [59] used E605 to kill her husband and her father-in-law. She also unintentionally poisoned Annie Hahman (intending to kill her mother Eva Ruh).

Dichlorvos or DDVP (2, 2-dychlorovynil-dimethyl-phosphate) is an organophosphate used as an insecticide. Its actions and symptoms are similar to those of other acetylcholinesterase inhibitors. He Tiandai [101] a carer poisoned He Yanzhu, a 70-year-old woman at the victim's home in Guandong Province, China. She administered sleeping pills and dichlorvos in soup, then injected the soup into the victim's stomach and hip. As the victim was dying, He Tiandai strangled her with a piece of rope.

Lead

A natural substance, galena, a lead sulphide ore, is heated to yield metallic lead which is heavy and fusible. It may take the form of inorganic lead salts or organic lead compounds such as tetraethyl. Lead acetate is an inorganic salt of lead combined with acetic acid which was in the past known as 'sugar of lead'. In antiquity, lead was used in jewellery, for making dishes, and as fishing weights and was also known as a poison. Today lead may be used for example in paints for boats and cars, mirror backing, as a PVC stabiliser, progressively effective hair dye, roof 'flashing', lead crystal and ceramic glazes.

Lead may be absorbed by the gastrointestinal tract if swallowed, and by the respiratory tracts if inhaled. About 15–20% of lead taken orally is retained in the body with the rest being excreted in faeces. Carried through the body in red blood cells, lead is deposited in bones, teeth, kidneys and liver. It binds to the suphydril groups of bodily proteins and also acts with carboxyl and phosphory groups, damaging cell metabolism. Lead poisoning affects the gastrointestinal tract, nervous system and kidneys. Symptoms may include headache, tetchiness, tiredness and gum discolouration. Severe poisoning leads to blindness, emaciation, kidney damage, convulsions and eventually paralysis and death.

After standing trail at the Old Bailey, London, Louisa Taylor [18] was hanged for using 'sugar of lead' to murder her friend Mary Ann Tregillis with whom she was staying.

Mercuric Chloride

Mined in countries where volcanoes have been active, mercury, a metallic element, is usually found combined with sulphur in the form of red mercuric sulphide (cinnabar) or in its metallic form as quicksilver. While cinnabar and quicksilver are naturally occurring forms, many other forms of mercury exist. Mercuric chloride is one of these, being an inorganic salt, which in past times was also known as sublimate of mercury.

Mercury and its salts were used medicinally by the ancients in China and in India, although its possible curative properties were not explored in the West until much later. Mercury and chalk (grey powder) or mercuric chloride (calomel) has been used as a laxative. Mercuric oxide was an antiseptic, and cinnabar was used to treat syphilis. Its past use in hat manufacturing is said by some to have led to the term, 'mad as a hatter' owing to the supposed effect of mercury on the mental state of these workers. Traditional barometers and thermometers also use mercury.

Mercuric chloride has itself had various past uses. It has been employed as an anti-bacterial agent. As a precipitant of abortion, it was causing fatalities as late as 1934. In the 1950s, it was introduced as an anti-cancer agent for the bowel but its ill effects have led to its being no longer used.

Taken orally, about 2 gm. of mercuric chloride can be lethal, while an intravenous injection of only 97 mg. can kill. In homicidal cases, the chosen administration is by mouth although its metallic taste has to be disguised. Its corrosive action causes the mouth and throat to become pale and very painful. Other symptoms include excessive salivation, vomiting about fifteen minutes after the substance has been taken, cramp in the limbs, abdominal pain and diarrhoea. Mercuric chloride is excreted by the kidneys where it causes damage, by the salivary glands where it creates irritation and salivation, and by the large intestine where it may cause ulceration. After about 24 h, ulcers may form on the gums, and the teeth may loosen.

In England, for financial gain, Mary Bateman [1] murdered a gullible acquaintance Rebecca Perigo with mercuric chloride (and arsenic).

Thallium

A soft, white metallic element, thallium produces a green line in the light spectrum, hence its name, 'thallos' being Greek for 'green shoot'. Its various forms include thallium sulphate, and oxide and bromide salts of thallium. For a time, thallium salts were used for ringworm of the scalp because they caused hair loss making it possible to better treat the affected surface. More recently thallium salts have been used in the manufacture of dye, paint, window glass and optical lenses, and in ant bait, and rat poison.

Thallous salts are readily absorbed from the mucous membranes of the mouth and gastrointestinal tract, as well as from the skin. The metal accumulates in the muscles, kidneys and spleen, and to a lesser extent, the hair and skin. Thallium is excreted in urine for up to 2 months after it has been taken. One of the most toxic of metals, thallium is odourless, tasteless and colourless, so cannot be detected in food or drink if used for homicidal poisoning. It has been detected in the remains of a homicide victim even after cremation.

For an adult, the minimum lethal dose is about 800 mg. of thallium sulphate. For a person weighing 70 kg., this represents 12 mg. per kg., of body weight. In its action, thallium competes with the body's potassium at enzyme active centres. At certain stages in the course of poisoning, thallium can resemble poisoning by arsenic, lead, mercury or carbon monoxide.

Acute symptoms include waves of severe abdominal pain, vomiting, diarrhoea and haemorrhage. Proteins are passed in the urine and only very small amount of urine are excreted. Bodily extremities become very painful so that even the pressure of a bedsheet is intolerable. Delirium, convulsions and coma follow. Circulatory collapse and respiratory failure may occur 20–40 h after symptoms first appear. Chronic symptoms show effects mainly on the nervous system. Nerves serving the hands and feet become inflamed. Power to control movement is lost, the face becomes paralysed, squinting develops. Eye pupils become widely dilated. Eruptions appear on the skin, and the palms of the hands and soles of the feet take on a horn-like quality. Hair loss becomes noticeable about 20 days after the initial dose. Appetite loss, vomiting and stomach pains develop.

Austrian Martha Marek [53] killed her husband Emil, her daughter, a relative Susanne Lowenstein, and a lodger using thallium for which in 1938, she was guillotined. In England, 23-year-old Graham Young [68] murdered work colleagues, Bob Egle and Fred Biggs using thallium (having previously been released from a secure hospital for poisoning his step mother). In Florida, in 1988, George Trepal [77] introduced thallium into bottles of Coca-Cola that had been purchased by a neighbouring family with whom he had had various disagreements, killing family member Peggy Carr.

Potassium Chloride

Potassium is a metallic chemical element which was first isolated from potash (the ashes of plants), hence its name. The chemical compound potassium chloride is odourless and either white or colourless. Easily dissolved in water, it has a salty taste. Potassium chloride is used in medicine and in food processing. It is also causes cardiac arrest as one of the cocktail of three drugs used in judicial lethal injections in some states of the US.

When nurse Orville Lynn Majors [79] worked at the Vermillion Country Hospital in Indiana in from 1993 to 1994, deaths of patients increased so exponentially that the hospital management became suspicious and suspended his licence to practice. Following a criminal investigation, and the exhumation of several patients, it was found that six bodies contained potassium chloride. In 1997, Majors was arrested and charged with these six murders for which he was sentenced to imprisonment.

Sodium Chloride

Sodium is a soft, silvery metallic element. Sodium chloride (salt) is a compound of sodium and chloride combining to form white crystals. As well as its use in cooking, salt is used as in cleaning and in de-icing. In the body, sodium chlorine has functions various function, for example helping to maintain the right levels of blood pressure and hydration. Ingesting too much sodium chloride can be harmful, produce symptoms of irritation to the gastrointestinal tract, vomiting, difficulty breathing, convulsions and ultimately causing death (Rowe et al. 2009, p. 639).

In New York State, Lacey Spears [96] used salt administered in heavy concentrations through a stomach feeding tube to gradually poison and kill her son Garnett-Paul Spears, aged 5 years. Projecting herself on various social media as a caring mother battling with her son's illness, she seems to have finally killed the child when worried that he might reveal that she was creating his illness.

Other Poisons

Carbon Monoxide

Carbon monoxide is present in coal gas, so-called town gas (from burning buildings and furniture) and in some car exhaust fumes. A colourless, odourless and tasteless gas, it is absorbed by the lungs into the bloodstream. A fatal dose is represented in breathing an atmosphere of one-tenth of 1% of carbon monoxide for 3 h, or a higher concentration for a shorter duration. Within this period, the carbon monoxide molecules outnumber the body's red blood cells by 4000 billion to one, affecting about half of the red blood cells so that there would be insufficient oxygen getting round the body to sustain life.

More precisely the action of the poison relates to the fact that haemoglobin of the red blood cells has about 250–300 times the affinity for carbon monoxide than has oxygen. As a result, in the lungs, haemoglobin combines with carbon monoxide instead of oxygen, effectively preventing the transportation of oxygen round the body as oxyhaemoglobin and depriving body tissues of oxygen. The gas affects the ganglia (clusters of nerve cells) at the base of the brain and can destroy parts of it, impairing mental faculties so that the individual is unaware of anything being wrong.

Symptoms of carbon monoxide poisoning can include the skin becoming cherry red, headache, dizziness, weakness, nausea and increased rate of breathing and heartbeat. Collapse, coma, respiratory failure and death follow. A patient suffering carbon monoxide poisoning is given a mixture of oxygen and 5% carbon dioxide to inhale as soon as possible; otherwise, artificial respiration is given in fresh air.

In England, Reginald Hinks [48] murdered his elderly father-in-law using carbon monoxide (in coal gas) by first knocking him unconscious then putting the old man's head in the gas oven. In depression-hit New York City in 1933, a group of men conspired to murder an Irish alcoholic Mike Malloy having taken out life insurance on him. The group were grocer Dan Keisberg [47], bar owner Tony Marino, bartender Joseph Murphy, hit man Anthony Bastone, undertaker Francis Pasqua, taxi driver Hersey Green and Dr. Frank Manzella. After various farcical attempts to kill Malloy, the conspirators eventually poisoned him with carbon monoxide in his bedroom, passing a hose from a gas fitting down his throat. Of the perpetrators, one was shot in a dispute, four were executed and three served prison sentences.

Chloroform

A volatile, heavy, colourless liquid with a pungent slightly sweet odour, chloroform was discovered in 1831 by Liebig. It is a compound of chlorine, carbon and hydrogen and mixes with alcohol or ether. In the past, one or two drops of chloroform were taken to ease sea sickness. Applied to the skin as a liniment, it was used to sooth rheumatic pain. It is also used as a solvent for fatty substances in various chemical processes. As a vapour, chloroform induces drowsiness in small doses (and unconsciousness in larger amounts) and was first employed as an anaesthetic by Sir James Young Simpson in 1847. Later, it was administered to ease pain in childbirth and to induce unconsciousness in surgery although it is now used for neither purpose.

Taken by mouth, chloroform is absorbed by the gastrointestinal tract. As a vapour, it is absorbed by the lungs and distributed into the bloodstream. Chloroform can sometimes kill quickly and suddenly after a very small dose by stopping the heart. One of its actions is to make the heart highly sensitive to the bodily hormone adrenalin, so that too much chloroform can lead to heart failure brought about by the body's own adrenalin secretion. It can also cause respiratory arrest. Death can sometimes occur several days after chloroform has been taken owing to damage to the liver, heart and especially the kidneys. To treat a chloroform overdose, oxygen and 5% carbon dioxide is inhaled which helps to clear the chloroform from the bloodstream.

French dentist Dr. Etienne Deschamps [23] after several times stupefying then sexually abusing 12-year-old Juliette Deitsh with chloroform, killed her with the substance. In England, Roger Cooper and his brother [99] murdered Roger's lover Sameena Imam using chloroform in 2015.

Acids

Acids have certain identifying properties, for example being able to neutralise alkalis, and are usually corrosive. Among mineral or inorganic acids are sulphuric and nitric acids, both of which have been used to poison. As might be expected, homicidal poisoning with acid is rare given that if it is administered orally the victim is likely to realise that they are consuming something harmful.

Nitric Acid

Nitric acid is a fuming liquid that is either colourless or very nearly so. Past uses include wart removal because of its strong corrosive action. In very dilute form it has been used in vegetable bitters, and for certain forms of diarrhoea.

Almost as soon as the acid is swallowed, it causes intense pain and vomiting. The vomit contains blood from which the water has been lost, remnants of food and bits of mucus, and has the appearance of coffee grounds. In the mouth gather pieces of tissue and foaming mucus which is white or bloodstained and later becomes yellow or brown. Being a powerful oxidising agent, nitric acid reacts with the protein of organic matter to form trinitrophenol. Nitrogen monoxide is given off and organic matter is turned yellow, leading to discolouration of body tissue and sometimes clothing. As gas is released, the stomach becomes distended and the individual belches to get rid of the gas. Collapse follows and suffocation may be caused by the irritant fumes. A fatal dose is about 30 ml. Although individuals have recovered after 60 ml.

In London, Israel Lipski [19] was convicted of sexually assaulting then murdering fellow lodging house tenant Miriam Angel by forcefully pouring nitric acid down her throat. Discovered by police hiding under Miriam's bed with acid burns around his mouth, Lipski had seemingly tried to kill himself with the same substance.

Hydrochloric Acid

Hydrochloric acid is a solution of hydrogen chloride in water. A powerful mineral acid, it is colourless but has a strong pungent odour. In the past is was called 'spirit of salts' owing to it being produced in medieval times from rock salt and green vitriol and later from common salt and sulfuric acid. In industry, it is used in making vinyl chloride for PVC plastic and other materials. It has uses in cleaning agents and other small scale applications. Both fumes from the solution and the liquid itself corrode human tissue damaging skin, respiratory organs and digestive organs.

Martha Rendell [34] of Perth, Australia, killed her stepson Arthur Morris [14] with hydrochloric acid. She was highly suspected by police of similarly murdering her stepdaughters Annie Morris (aged 7) and Olive Morris (aged 5). Her method was to give food or drink causing sore throat then 'treating' this with a solution of the 'spirit of salts' painted on the inside of the mouth, claiming that she was giving a treatment for diphtheria.

Paraquat

A commercially produced contact herbicide, Paraquat is used in agriculture and horticulture. Gramoxone is a concentrated solution of Paraquat, while Weedol is a granular preparation of the substance. When using Paraquat in farming and plant care, workers have to be careful to protect the eyes and skin. About a mouthful of Paraquat can prove fatal. It burns the throat, causes fibrosis of the lungs making breathing increasingly laborious, and attacks vital organs. About two teaspoons of Gramoxone taken in a single dose is likely to be fatal. Death is almost always delayed. If it occurs within a few days, it is likely to be owing to kidney damage. After 1–3 weeks, respiratory damage is the usual cause.

In England, Susan Barber [71] poisoned her husband with Gramoxone introduced into a steak and kidney pie for which in 1982, she was sentenced to life imprisonment.

Antifreeze

Antifreeze may be methanol or ethylene glycol. Methanol (also known as 'methyl alcohol') is colourless, smells slightly of alcohol, is soluble in water and has a burning taste. It is used in windshield cleaning solution, paint remover and gas-line antifreeze (which may be 95% methanol). A fatal dose is about 20–150 gm. In the body, methanol is oxidised to form the more toxic formaldehyde, which is further oxidised into formic acid. Symptoms appear between a few hours when the individual will appear drunk and have stomach pains, and 30 h when symptoms include excessive production of body acid, visual disturbances, blindness, seizures and coma, and eventually death (Trestrail 2007, pp. 111–114).

The compound, ethylene glycol (1,2 ethanol) is a viscous liquid that is odourless, sweet tasting and highly soluble in water. It is used in radiator antifreeze as well as in antifreeze products for heating and cooling systems. The fatal dose of 95% ethylene glycol is about 1.5 mL per kg of body weight.

In the body, the compound is oxidised into the more toxic oxalic acid which then combines with blood calcium to form crystals of calcium oxalate which can be found in the kidneys and in urine. Symptoms appear with in 4–12 h, the early symptoms being apparent drunkenness and possible gastritis and vomiting. After 4–12 h the individual experiences acidosis, hyperventilation, convulsion, heartbeat disturbances and coma and often kidney failure (Trestrail 2007, pp. 111–114).

In California, in 2000 after taking out life insurance on her fourth husband, Angelina Rodriguez [84] killed him with ethylene glycol-based 'green' antifreeze in his sports drink bottle. Arrested in 2001, and found guilty she was sentenced to death. In 2001 the boyfriend of Lynn Turner [88] (Randy Thompson) died and police investigations into the similar death of her former husband Glenn Turner convinced them that she had killed both with ethylene glycol-based antifreeze.

Found guilty in 2004 of Turner's murder, and in 2007 of Thompson's murder, Julia Lynn Turner died in prison in 2010. James Keown [91] a US radio reporter poisoned his wife Julie with antifreeze administered in her Gatorade in 2004 to get money from her life insurance. A check of his computer revealed searches for ethylene glycol poisoning. Stacey Castor [92] was sentenced to life imprisonment in 2009 for the second degree murder of her second husband David Castor with antifreeze apparently forcefully fed to him when he was too weak to resist.

N-Nitrosodimethylamine

N-Nitrosodimethylamine, also known as dimethylnitrosamine, is a semi-volatile organic chemical produced as by-product of several industrial processes. Water soluble and colourless, it has either a faint smell or no discernible odour. Symptoms of poisoning by *N*-Nitrosodimethylamine include headache, fever, vomiting, abdominal pain, nausea, diarrhoea, bleeding under the skin, and lethargy. The substance is harmful to the liver.

In September 1978, Steven Roy Harper [69] a jealous former boyfriend of Sandra Johnson introduced *N*-Nitrosodimethylamine to lemonade drinks at the Johnson home in Omaha, Nebraska. Harper had acquired the poison working at the University of Nebraska Medical Centre Eppley Cancer Center in March 1978, where it was used in the laboratory to induce cancer in mice for study. As a result of the poisoning Sandra's husband Duane and their 11-month-old son Chad Sheldon both died.

Conclusion

This chapter discussed elements, their compounds and derivatives and 'other poisons' in each case, looking at homicidal poisoners who had used these substances.

Suggested Activities

Consider several cases from the glossary of arsenic poisoning in different time periods. Note some possible reasons for the predominance use of arsenic as a criminal poison especially in the nineteenth and early twentieth centuries.

Key Texts

Emsley (2005) *The Elements of Murder: A History of Poison* Oxford, Oxford University Press

The book examines the elements of mercury, arsenic, antimony, lead and thallium, looking at their history and use in crime and taking into account the chemistry of these substances.

References

Emsley, J. (2005). *The elements of murder: a history of poison oxford*, Oxford University Press.

Farrell, M. (1989). Many Faced Poison. *Police Review*, 97(5032), 2022–2023.

Farrell, M. (1990). Arsenic queen of poisons. *Criminologist, 14*(4), 188–189.

Rowe, R. C., Sheskey, P. J. & Quinn, M. E. (Eds.) (2009). *Handbook of pharmaceutical excipients* (6th ed.). London: Pharmaceutical Press.

Trestrail, J. H. (2007). *Criminal poisoning: Investigational guide for law enforcement, toxicologists, forensic scientists and attorneys* (2nd ed.). Totowa, NJ: Humana Press.

Chapter 7
Poisoners and Their Characteristics

Introduction

Attempts to reach generalisations about any characteristics of poisoners have ranged from looking in detail at a small number of cases considered and analysing statistics involving many cases. Multiple poisoning provides useful insights into poisoning and may involve several people being killed at the same time (simultaneous poisoning), several people being killed one after the other over an extended period of time (serial poisoning). Cases of 'team poisoning' arise in which two or more perpetrators act together to poison a victim or victims. Whether poisoning is acute or chronic can shed light on the intentions of the poisoner.

Rowland's Twelve Cases

Seeking characteristics of poisoners, Rowland (1960) scrutinised twelve cases: Dr. William Palmer Dr. William [8], Dr. Edward Pritchard [12], Dr. George Lamsom [17], Louisa Taylor [18], and Adelaide Bartlett, Dr. Hawley Crippen [35], Ethel Major [49], Charlotte Bryant [51], Dorothea Waddingham [50], Louisa Merrifield [58], Arthur Ford [60], and Kenneth Barlow [63]. Chronologically, the examples range from the mid-18 hundreds when Palmer [8] was tried, to just before Rowland published, when Kenneth Barlow [63] was convicted. Male and female poisoners are discussed and the offenders come from various social backgrounds. However, Adelaide Bartlett was not convicted of poisoning her husband Edwin and his suicide remains a plausible explanation (Farrell 1994).

Rowland suggests several characteristics common to poisoners: an unfortunate married life, low educational level, failing to make their mark in life, vanity, childhood experience, lacking in sympathy and imagination, and great ruthlessness. Many of these suggestions are problematic. For example, the supposed

M. Farrell, *Criminology of Homicidal Poisoning*,
DOI 10.1007/978-3-319-59117-9_7

characteristic of low educational level is contradicted by several of Rowland's own examples who were physicians. The most credible suggestion is that of great ruthlessness. For example in some chronic poisonings, the perpetrator administers the substance knowing and witnessing its effects, suggesting cruelty, and perhaps an enjoyment of power over a victim (Farrell 1993).

Observations from Published Poisoning Cases

Drawing on published sources, Trestrail (2007) suggests that poisoners are: cunning, 'artistic' (being able to design and plan the murder in detail), cowardly (non-confrontational), childlike in their fantasy and avaricious (Ibid. pp. 50–52).

Where poisonings are carefully thought out and concealed, the attributes of 'cunning' and of being 'artistic' seem apt. Most poisonings avoid physical or mental confrontation because the victim is oblivious of their plight, unless exceptionally poison is administered forcibly as when Reginald Hinks [48] poisoned his father-in-law James Pullen with carbon monoxide from a domestic supply. Having childlike fantasies may apply to some poisoners such as nurse Genene Jones [74] who poisoned children then sought adulation by 'saving' them. But a fantasy life would also describe other criminals, for example burglars dreaming of wealth. Being avaricious is likely to fit poisoners whose motive is monetary gain, such as Frederick Seddon [37] but again, this applies to other crimes.

Trestrail's Typology

Trestrail (2007) proposes a categorisation of poisoners relating to the extent of their planning, and the specificity of their victims reflecting different motivations (Ibid. pp. 47–49). The typology comprises 'specific' or 'random' victim, and 'quickly' or 'carefully' planned administration of poison.

In 'types S' cases, a specific (S) victim is targeted and the motive tends to be: money (perhaps from life insurance), removing someone or something blocking a desired goal, jealousy, revenge and political motives such as assassination and terrorism. Group R cases involve a random (R) victim with motives of: sadism; egotistical belief in one's mental superiority; the desire to tamper; and boredom leading to seeking fun by challenging law enforcement. Within each of these broad groupings are two sub-groups (Ibid. pp. 47–49, 54).

Where victims are specific, the poisoning may be slowly planned with a carefully chosen poison (specific/slow); or quickly planned (specific/quick). If the victim is specific and the poisoning slowly planned, this would typically involve careful thought about the circumstances, the poison, and how it would be administered. Where the victim is specific but the planning quick the perpetrator would likely act in anger, seizing a readily available poison and administering it at an early opportunity.

With a random victim, the poisoning may be slowly planned with a carefully chosen poison (random/slow); or quickly planned (random/quick). In the 'random/slow' scenario, a perpetrator might introduce a carefully considered poison into a retail food or medicine in a store anticipating blackmailing the respective company, or may threaten terrorism. Should a victim be random and the planning quick, a perpetrator may act in anger, using a quickly available poison but lacing products such as food or drugs where the victims cannot be predicted.

Trestrail (2007) highlights deceptive, camouflaged poisonings which appear random but are in fact specific. Stella Nickell [75] for example killed her husband Bruce with cyanide, and tampered with over the counter pain killers on sale locally to make it appear that her husband had taken a contaminated product. In doing this she also caused the death of local bank manager Susan Snow (Ibid. pp. 22–23).

US Homicide Statistics

Here, we refer to Uniform Crime Reports (UCR) concerning the 'uniform' nature of the reporting documents across the various jurisdictions (Dobrin 2016, p. 6). In the US, 2014 UCR homicide data provides information on the gender, age and race of perpetrators. Much of this is found in 'Expanded Homicide Data, Table 3, Murder Offenders by Age, Sex, Race and Ethnicity, 2014'.(Federal Bureau of Investigation 2015). Some figures from this database are given below to provide context for discussing poison homicide. Comparisons are suggestive but limited because the general homicide data and the poison homicide figures cover different periods.

US Poisoning Statistics

An epidemiological study of poisonings in the US (Westveer et al. 1996) examined UCR data kept by the Department of Justice from 1980 to 1989. The reports submitted annually by police agencies across the US, provides victim and offender information for various crimes. It includes the month, year and state; victim information (gender, age, race/ethnicity); offender information (gender, age, race/ethnicity); classification of the poisonous agent (drug, non-drug, fume); relationship between offender and victim; and a classification of motive. In the decade covered, 202, 785 homicides were reported of which there were 292 cases of a single offender poisoning a single victim (14 poison cases per 10,000 homicides). Of the whole population, per million people, poisons averaged 1.47 per year. Westveer et al. (2004) repeated the earlier study on 1990–1999 data and found similar proportions.

Gender of Poisoners: Statistics

Homicide in General

Statistics for homicide in general show a clear male predominance in offenders. For example, FBI data 2014, UCR Crime in the US provides homicide data (Federal Bureau of Investigation 2015). If one looks at *all* reported offenders 63.1% were male, 8.4% were female and for 28.5% the gender was unknown. Of offenders *for whom gender is known*, 88.2% were male (Ibid.). As Brookman (2005) states, gender is especially important regarding homicide given that, 'males (more specifically men) are vastly over represented as both offenders and (albeit less dramatically) victims of homicide' (Ibid. p. 309).

Poison Homicide

In a database of 1026 cases in which the offender was convicted of homicidal poisoning most cases were from either the US (404) or the UK (255) with the remainder from many different regions (Trestrail 2007, pp. 56–57). Dates span from 339 B. C. E. to 2007 and are mainly from the twentieth century (Trestrail, personal communication, November 2016). Some 45% of the offenders were male and 39% female (in 16% of cases poisoner's gender was not recorded). In 420 instances there was more than one victim and of these cases, 46% were perpetrated by males and 43% by females (for 11% the gender was unknown). There was more than 1 offender in 120 of the 1026 cases and of these, 46% were male and 52% female (Trestrail 2007, pp. 56–61).

Watson (2004) analysed poison cases from Assizes Records and other sources in England and Wales from 1750 to 1914 and found that for 540 cases, 48.7% of those accused were male and 51.3% female. These figures correspond to the gender proportions in the nineteenth century population of England and Wales (Ibid. p. 45 and p. 46 Table 3). Regarding general homicide, men were three times as likely as women to commit murder, but when women did murder, they were far more likely than men to choose poison (Ibid. p. 45).

In the US, 1980–1989 UCR data (Westveer et al. 1996) suggest that twice as many poison offenders were male than were female.

If prior to the early twentieth century, female poisoning was more prevalent than male, it may relate to the difficulty for women obtaining a divorce when marriage failed, and opportunity to administer poison would be easier when women traditionally prepared and served meals (or in middle class households supervised the process). As Watson (2004) observes, 'many of the stimuli to murder experienced by the Victorian poor have been removed' (Ibid. p. 217). She continues, 'Divorce is readily available, female employment opportunities have expanded, infant mortality rates are low, child deaths are investigated aggressively, insurance companies use sophisticated techniques to root out fraud, and national social welfare systems offer a safety net to those who fall on hard times' (Ibid.). It appears that, more recently the number of men poisoners equals or exceeds women perhaps because previous female incentives have receded, but there is nothing like the male preponderance associated with homicide in general.

Gender of Poisoners: Illustrative Cases

There is no evidence for particular female adeptness for poisoning. Certainly there are husband murders like Edith Carew [26], Maria Groesbeek [67] and Marie Hilley [70]. But there are also wife killers such as Kenneth Barlow [63], Eugène Chantrelle [16] and George Chapman [29]. Women serial poisoners include Mary Bateman [1] and Mary Cotton [14]. But equally, one can cite male serial poisoners such as Graham Young [68] and Dr. Harold Shipman [81].

Against the deviousness of Amy Archer-Gillighan [41], who killed her nursing home patients for financial gain, can be set the cunning of Dr. William Palmer [8] executed for murdering his horseracing companion. Cordelia Botkin [28] showed the foresight to plan murder at a distance by sending arsenic impregnated chocolates through the mail. Similarly, Adoph Hofrichter [36] jealous of the promotion of infantry colleagues, mailed cyanide as a supposed aphrodisiac to twelve of them.

In a traditional food-preparing role, Susan Barber [71] added Paraquat to her husband's steak and kidney pie. Charlotte Bryant [51] put arsenic in her husband's Oxo drink. Marie Lafarge [4] mailed cakes mixed with arsenic to her husband when he was away from home, administering further doses to kill him on his return. Corned beef was dosed with strychnine by Ethel Major [49] to kill her truck driver husband. But there are also examples of men poisoning food or drink although not necessarily fare that they have prepared. Richard Brinkley [33] killed the landlord and landlady of an acquaintance with cyanide laced stout. Using aconite impregnated Dundee cake Dr. George Lamson [17] murdered his brother-in-law. Jean Pierre Vaquier [45] left strychnine in Bromo salts that he knew would be drunk by his lover's husband. In China, Wei Entan [87], aggrieved at being jilted by a married woman, gave her children rat poisoned oranges and popcorn.

Age of Poisoners: Statistics

Homicide in General

FBI data for 2014, UCR Crime in the US provides homicide information indicating that of offenders *for whom age is known*, offending peaks in several age bands between the ages of 17 and 35 years (Federal Bureau of Investigation 2015).

Poison Homicide

Turning to poisoning homicide, analysis of the 1980–1989 UCR data (Westveer et al. 1996) indicated that the highest number of offenders was in the age band 20–34 years. (There were 292 cases in the 1 perpetrator 1 victim total).

Age of Poisoners: Illustrative Cases

Many poisonings it appears are perpetrated by individuals in their 20s and 30s as is evident in many cases cited in this book. But the age range takes in much younger and much older perpetrators too. Relatively youthful poisoners include Graham Young [68] who was aged 15 years when sent to a secure psychiatric prison in 1962 for poisoning family members. His better known poisonings occurred after his release (in 1971) when he killed two work colleagues with thallium when he was still only 24 years old. Ryan Furlough [86] was a 17-year-old school student when he killed his friend Benjamin Vassilev with cyanide in a soda drink.

Among comparatively older poisoners Quaker John Tawell [5] was 61 when he used prussic acid in a bottle of 'stout' to kill Sarah Lawrence his mistress. Irish physician Dr. Philip Cross [20] was 62 when he added arsenic to his wife Laura's sodium bromide medication, killing her so that he could marry his lover Effie Skinner. Mary Wilson [64] was aged 64 when she used phosphorus beetle poison to kill Ernest Wilson, her third husband. US Neuroscientist Dr. Robert Ferrante [97] was also 64 when he poisoned his wife Dr. Autumn Klein with cyanide.

Race of Poisoners: Statistics

Homicides in General

Administrative race categories have been criticised for being inconsistent (Phillips and Bowling 2012, p. 372). FBI data of 2014, UCR Crime in the US provides information on race categories of 'white', 'black' and 'other races'. Where the *race of the offender was known*, 53.0% were black, 44.7% were white, and 2.3% were of 'other races'. Offender's race was unknown for 4132 of 13,897 offenders (Federal Bureau of Investigation 2015).

Poison Homicide

Comparable figures relating to poison murder do not appear to be available, but there are relative figures on race and poisoning in the 1980–1989 UCR data

(Westveer et al. 1996). These indicate that: offender and victim were usually of the same race; if the victim was white, the offender was usually male; and if the victim was black, the offender could equally be male or female. (Most victims were white; there were equal numbers of white female and white male victims; and twice as many black victims were male than female).

Race of Poisoners: Illustrative Cases

Poisoners tend to be the same race as their victims. Spouse murders and murders of relatives are common poison killings, tending to be within the same racial groups. Examples of same-race (Asian) homicides are the cyanide poisoning of Wayan Salihin by Jessica Wongso [100] in Indonesia; and

Sadamichi Hirasawa [56] in Japan tricking members of bank staff into taking cyanide so that he could rob the premises. Poisoning where perpetrator and victim have different racial origins is less usual, an example being Roger and David Cooper [99], both White, chloroforming Roger Cooper's Asian lover Sameena Imam.

Occupation/Social Background of Poisoners: Illustrative Cases

Medical and Related Occupations

Physicians, nurses, managers of nursing homes, dentists and medical students—all of these occupations have produced poisoners. Physicians can put themselves in a position to murder and make detection difficult (Simpson 1978). A doctor has access to potentially lethal drugs as well as knowledge of the symptoms of poisoning and how these might be passed off as disease or illness. Dr. Henry Clark [39] aided by Augusta Fullam used this knowledge to present their victim's death from arsenic poisoning as heatstroke.

Both doctors and nurses interpret symptoms and are often present at times of a patient's deterioration, when drugs used to ease pain or for surgical procedures can be abused to kill. Japanese nurse Daisuke Mori [85] used a vecuronium bromide overdose to kill patient Yukiko Shimoyama at a clinic in Sendai. Assessing the cause of death and completing the death certificate being part of a physician's duties, can also be abused. Dr. Philip Cross [20] poisoned his wife with arsenic then got a young, inexperienced doctor to concur with his diagnosis of typhoid. Murder by medical personnel extends beyond killing patients. Anaesthiologist Dr. Carl Coppolino [66] injected his wife with succinylcholine chloride. The notion that there is a preponderance of medical poisoners is supported by Trestrail's (2007) analysis of 1026 cases in which 6% were physicians, and 4% were nurses (ibid. p. 57–58).

Increasingly as the population in many Western countries live longer, the role of carers perhaps working for an agency is increasing. Carers have intimate access to clients as with He Tiandai [101] in China who poisoned an elderly client with sleeping pills and dichlorvos. With training, carers may also supervise their clients taking prescribed medication and record this, perhaps for clients with memory impairing conditions. This opens the possibility of poisoning to members of the rapidly growing (and sometimes poorly governed) work force. For example, a carer might conceal poisoning by suggesting that a client inadvertently took an overdose of a medication or mistakenly took another drug.

Other Occupations with Access to Poisons

It is not only medical professionals, who have access to potential poisons. Arthur Ford [60], General Office Manager of a manufacturing chemist stole cantharides from the stores to administer to a secretary, thinking that it was an aphrodisiac. Farmer Daniel Bondeson [83] who killed Walter Morrill a fellow church worshiper with arsenic likely used an out of date agricultural product from his own or another local farm.

Domestic Service and Hospitality Occupations

Where occupations involve preparing food and drink for others, poisoning becomes possible, as in the days when domestic service in an employer's household was prevalent. Anna Zwanziger [2] took domestic posts in different parts of Germany, murdering her employers. Housekeeper Louisa Merrifield [53] ended her employer's life with phosphorus.

In hospitality businesses where interactions with others is less regular, such as in public houses, bars and hotels, poisoning is less likely than in the case of a household employee. Nevertheless, Jean Vaquier [45] himself a hotel worker poisoned the husband of his lover in the couple's public house. In India, K.D. Kempanna [94] who killed temple devotees with cyanide worked as a domestic help at several places in the Bangalore suburbs but the killing appears to have been unconnected with this.

The Range of Occupations

While some work presents particular opportunity for poisoning, poisoners also come from many occupations. Sales people who have poisoned include insurance broker Henri Girrard [42] who killed his fellow worker and a widow for financial gain. Insurance seller Edward Black poisoned his wife with arsenic, fleeing the district to try to avoid detection. Hoover dealer Reginald Hinks [44] gassed his father-in-law. Military poisoners include Marcus Marymont [65] of the US Air Force, and Austrian Army officer Adolph Hofrichter [36]. Walter Horsford [27] was a farmer as was Daniel Bondeson [83]. Eugène Chantrelle [16] worked as a French teacher, Johann Hoch [32] was a packing house worker, and Sadamachi Hirasawa [56] was an artist. Marie Hilley [70] worked as a secretary, and Louisa Taylor a milliner [18]. Wife killer Herbert Armstrong was a lawyer [43].

Multiple Homicides and Multiple Poison Homicides

Multiple Homicides in General

Estimating the number of multiple murders is problematic. Connections between several apparently different and separate unsolved murders may go unrecognised. Ressler et al. (1988) estimate that in the US between 30 and 100 individual multiple murderers may be active at any one time. While there is disagreement how many death constitute 'multiple homicide' (Rappaport 1988), a helpful distinction may be made between 'mass homicide' and 'serial homicide' (Lester 1995).

Mass homicide involves instances when 'multiple victims are killed in a single episode and in the same geographic location' (Brookman 2005, p. 211) for example in a mass shooting. Serial homicides are ones which, 'occur repetitively over an extended period' (Ibid.). A suggested minimum period is more than 30 days (Holmes and Holmes 2001), but it may be much longer. Serial killings are associated with a period of 'cooling off', distinguishing them from mass killing. Briefly, serial murder is, 'the unlawful killing of two or more victims by the same perpetrator(s), in separate incidents comprising a series' (Behavioural Analysis Unit 2005, pp. 8–9).

Daniszewska (2017) argues that the number of serial murder killers and victims has declined. For example, early estimates of 200 serial murders in the US fell to 100 at the beginning of the twenty-first century. Improvements in DNA research and fingerprint matching to specimens in computer databases may have precipitated this (Ibid. p. 13).

Mitchell (1997) provides an integrated model of serial murder. It draws together pathological foundations (such as interacting biological, family and sociocultural factors) and developmental consequences (for example possible sexual fantasies/dysfunction). Among typologies is that of Fox and Levin (2011), who distinguish those driven by power, revenge, loyalty, benefit or terror. The most common type is thought to be the serial killer thirsting for power and control who uses force (Ibid. pp. 23–26).

Multiple Poisoning

Mass poisonings have occurred in exceptional circumstances perhaps involving a cult suicide pact, or during wartime. In more 'conventional' poisonings of more than one person, the numbers of victims tend to be fewer than in other mass homicides (by shooting for example). The term, 'simultaneous poisonings' might be more appropriate for such cases.

Serial poisoning can allow the poisoners to pass off individual deaths in different ways, such as by natural causes. Done on a domestic scale, as with the poisoning of successive spouses it can raise suspicion, but carried out in a medical context, serial poisoning can go undetected for long periods. Profiling can be useful with non-poisoning killers (including serial killers) where victims and the circumstances of the murder can be examined and compared with other cases or with possibly related instances Alison (2005). However, profiling is unavailable with poisoners (including serial poisoners) where no one is aware that murder has occurred. Below we examine briefly examples of simultaneous poisoning, and more fully instances of serial poisoning.

Simultaneous Poisoning

Simultaneous poisoning involves more than one victim being poisoned in a single episode, and in the same location. Such poisonings were perpetrated by Arthur Ford [60] by doctoring confections with cantharides, leading to the deaths of two secretaries. Arthur Deveureux [31] poisoned his wife Beatrice and twin sons at the same time and disposed of their bodies in a trunk, which he had stored in a warehouse. Richard Brinkley [33] intending to kill a potential witness to forgery Reginald Parker, instead inadvertently and simultaneously killed Parker's visiting landlord and wife. In order to rob a bank in Japan, Sadamichi Hirasawa [56] poisoned several tellers by giving them cyanide, pretending that he was an official issuing precautionary medication.

Reflecting the problems for the perpetrator in avoiding detection in simultaneous poisonings, it is notable that Arthur Ford did not intend to kill but to sexually arouse a secretary whom he found attractive, thinking that cantharides was an aphrodisiac. Deveureux disposed of the bodies of his three victims. Brinkley intended to kill one person, not two. Hirasawa had no connection with the bank employees whom he killed.

Serial Poisoning

General Points

Serial poisoners tend to kill people whom they know whereas other serial killers tend to attack strangers. Trestrail (2007) drawing on a database of 1026 cases in which the offender was convicted of homicidal poisoning, found that in 59% of cases involve one victim but in the remaining 41% of cases, there were 'multiple victims' (Ibid. p. 59). Poisoning tends to be an invisible crime if death is not considered suspicious and can be mistaken for natural causes. Where a perpetrator has evaded suspicion once, further killings become possible. As Kelleher and Kelleher (1998) point out, female serial killers acting alone tend to choose poisoning as their weapon (see also, Holmes and Holmes 2010).

Cases examined by Trestrail (2007) suggest that about one in ten poison homicides (120 cases of 1026) involve multiple perpetrators. Examples are Mary Creighton and Everett Applegate [52] who poisoned Everett's wife Ada; the group of seven men including Dan Keisberg [47] who gassed Mike Malloy with carbon monoxide; and Sarah Anne Pearson and Agnes Black [30] who poisoned Alice Pearson with strychnine.

Where there are multiple perpetrators, there may also be multiple victims (Trestrail 2007, p. 60).

Where two or more people act together to poison they may have separate grievances against different people. Lovers Dr. Henry Clark and Augusta Fullam [39] each wanting to be rid of their respective spouse, colluded in poisoning Augusta's husband Edward.

Medical Serial Poisoners

It is plausibly maintained that medicine has 'thrown up more serial killers than all the other professions put together, with nursing a close second' (Kinnell 2000). Medical professionals have the opportunity to acquire drugs, access to patients for treatment, and often enjoy the trust of the local community. When medics become poisoners, it may be difficult to detect that anything untoward is happening for a considerable period of time. It has been suggested that the motivation of those who kill others in their care relates to 'issues of power and control as well as a fundamental objectification of people' (Hough and McCorkle 2017, p. 158).

In nursing homes, especially for elderly residents, where deaths are expected from time to time, nurses and nursing home managers can exploit this. Amy Archer-Gilligan [41] killed four of her nursing home patients. Dorothea Waddingham [50] in England used morphine to kill her patients Louisa Baguley and Ada Baguley (Louisa's daughter). In Norway, Arnfinn Nessett [72] killed 21 of his nursing home residents over several years using succinylcholine chloride.

Where individuals are in hospitals the fact that death is sometimes expected can be abused. Dr. Michael Swango [80] killed four patients with arsenic and may have murdered many more. Nurse Orville Lynn Majors [79] used potassium chloride to kill six patients at Vermillion County Hospital. Nurse Victorino Chua [98] was convicted of arranging overdoses of insulin to two patients.

In non-hospital settings, Dr. Edward Pritchard [12] used aconite (and antimony) to poison Mary Jane Taylor his wife, and Jane Cowan his mother-in-law. Dr. Marcel Petiot [55], in occupied France, poisoned 24 people over several years, using cyanide. At different times, Dr. Neill Cream [22] gave strychnine to four London prostitutes, killing all of them. In the cases of Petiot and Cream had anyone been able to detect the early killings there was a signature to the murders which might have aided detection. For example Cream selected prostitutes, tended not to be present when the death occurred, and used cyanide.

Other Serial Poisoners

Some serial poisoners killed their spouse (and other relatives including their children). Johan Hoch [32] poisoned his wife Julia Walcker-Hoch with arsenic and may have murdered other wives. Mary Wilson [64] killed both her second and third husbands with elemental phosphorus. Martha Marek [53] of Vienna, used thallium to kill her husband Emil Marek, her daughter Ingeborg, a relative Susanne Lowenstein, and a lodger Frau Kittenberger. Nannie Doss [61] in Oklahoma used arsenic to poison five husbands, her mother, two sisters, two children, and a nephew. Christa Lehman [59] in Germany employed E605 to kill her husband Karl and Valentin Lehman her father-in-law, also inadvertently poisoning her friend Annie Hamann.

Domestic service especially if itinerant can allow serial poisoning. Anna Zwanziger [2] worked in different parts of Germany providing opportunity to poison with arsenic employers or their spouses Frau Glaser, Judge Grohmann and Frau Gebhardt. Obsessed with poisons, Graham Young [68] used thallium to murder two work colleagues.

Theory: Serial Poisoning

Differential reinforcement theory (Jeffrey 1965), in which criminal behaviour and its frequency is determined by the positive or negative consequences it creates could apply to serial poisoning. Where a perpetrator is not caught yet gains financially or otherwise from the death of their victim, this might ‘reinforce’ the crime. Second attempts at poisoning where an earlier one has ‘succeeded’ could be explained in this way as with Lynn Turner [88] poisoning her former husband and later her boyfriend.

Control theory seems applicable to the so-called 'life course' studies and careers of delinquency (or its rejection) in the light of social bonds and other influences over time (Laub and Sampson 2003). This may aid understanding of a 'career' of serial poisoning where refinements are made and the perpetrator becomes increasingly adept at avoiding detection, as with Dr. Harold Shipman [81].

Labelling theory (Becker 1963) may apply. A poisoner may witness accounts of their crimes in the mass media and gradually shape their offending according to these depictions. Such an individual is not directly confronted by others' views and reactions but experiences it secretly through the media and through what others around them unsuspectingly say. Perhaps in this way, someone such as Graham Young come to see themselves as 'a poisoner' encouraging this deviant identity.

Team Poisoning

Team Poisoners

In the team murder perpetrated by brothers Roger and David Copper [99] Roger appeared to be the potential beneficiary of the crime in avoiding exposure of his affair with his lover Sameena. Yet his brother was jointly involved in planning, carrying out, and concealing the crime. The murder by Dan Keisberg [47] and six accomplices involved them acting together to poison Mike Malloy with carbon monoxide gas. Lovers Mary Creighton and Everett Applegate [52] were jointly responsible for poisoning Everett's wife Ada with arsenic. In colonial India, Dr. Henry Clark and Augusta Fullam [39] colluded to poison Augusta's husband Edward with arsenic, which Clarke suggested using in order to mimic symptoms of heatstroke. Having sent the poison to Augusta to administer to her husband, Clarke then attended Edward and treated him for this fictitious heatstroke after which the victim soon died.

Theory—Team Poisoning

Work on subculture (Cohen 1957) may illuminate team poison homicide, where the offenders mutually mitigate the meaning of the deviant behaviour. Such poisonings are rare, reflecting that poisoning is typically chosen for its secrecy and therefore acting with another is anathema. But where team poisoning does occur, mitigation seems plausible.

Roger and David Cooper may have down-played the seriousness and risk of the crime through believing that acting together, they minimised the chances of being detected. In the murder of Mike Malloy it appears that the group who killed him mutually encouraged each other, perhaps believing in safety in numbers. Mary

Creighton and Everett Applegate may have diminished the gravity of their actions by planning together. Everett had discovered that Mary had previously been accused of poisoning but acquitted so any mitigation may have been tinged with threat. (Mary administered the arsenic). Possibly, Clark and Fullam had mitigating discussions but additionally, there was the joint motive of wanting to be rid of their respective spouses so that they could be together.

Acute and Chronic Poisoning

Distinguishing Acute and Chronic Poisoning

Acute poisoning aims to murder the victim quickly while chronic poisoning kills slowly over a longer period. With poisons such as arsenic the effect is more dependent on the dose than is the case with some other poisons as arsenic can kill quickly or slowly. Other poisons are associated with acute action. Symptoms of cyanide poisoning usually appear within a few minutes. Strychnine too generally has a rapid effect often producing violent symptoms shortly after being consumed.

Acute Poisoning

Many poisonings are acute, death taking place soon after the poison has been administered. A single or few administrations of poison over a short period may be considered less likely to attract suspicion than many small administrations over a longer duration. Other situational constraints may be placed on the perpetrator.

Lakvir Singh [93] in putting aconite in a curry to be eaten by her former lover Lakhvinder Cheema and his fiancé needed the poison to act quickly in a single dose. No longer able to stay with Cheema regularly as she had done previously, Lakvir's access to his home was now limited and she could not expect to poison over a protracted period. Roger and David Cooper [99] chloroformed to death Roger Cooper's lover Sameena Imam to prevent her from revealing the relationship between herself and Roger. Intending to dispose of Sameena Imam's body, the brothers had to use a quick acting poison.

Chronic Poisoning

Chronic poisoning may be used to suggest that the victim has been unwell for a long time so that their death is expected. Major Herbert Armstrong [43] appears to have administered arsenic to his wife Katherine until she was admitted to a sanatorium where she began to recover, then continued the poisoning after she was discharged until she died. Cause of death was initially certified as heart problems.

In other instances, chronic poisoning suggests sadistic motives. In Perth, Australia, Martha Rendell [34] swabbed the mouth of her step son 14-year-old Arthur Morris with hydrochloric acid over an extended period (as a supposed treatment for sore throat) leading to a lingering death. Sadistic motives were attributed to Graham Young [68] who kept a diary detailing the sufferings of his victims.

In one sense chronic poisoning is the serial poisoning of the same person over time, so the same theories may apply. Differential reinforcement theory (Jeffrey 1965), in which criminal behaviour and its frequency is determined by its positive or negative consequences is an example. Control theory (Laub and Sampson 2003) relating to careers of delinquency in the light of social bonds and other influences over time may be relevant to chronic poisoning where refinements are made and the perpetrator becomes increasingly adept at avoiding detection. Labelling theory (Becker 1963) may apply as the chronic poisoner hears concerned onlookers debating what might be wrong with the victim, secretly shaping the poisoner's sense of identity accordingly.

Theories of Poisoning in General

We can now revisit some theories of poisoning in general. It has been suggested that offending is associated with delays in the development of moral reasoning. When opportunity to offend arises, an individual then lacks the reasoning to resist the temptation (Kohlberg 1978). This can apply to poisoning in that it involves calculated planning and reasoning.

Rational choice theory (Clarke 1992) may help explain factors which influence decisions to commit or not to commit criminal activities. An example of 'controlling facilitators' would be limiting the sale and purchase of poisons and tightening rules for death certification to deter medical poisoning.

Feminism and a 'gendered' view of crime (e.g., Gelsthorpe and Morris 1982) may have relevance for homicidal poisoning. Views about female perpetrators seem sometimes to have been based on stereotypes. The idea that poisoning is a predominantly female crime is not sustainable, certainly not in the modern day. In some poison trials, gender may have had an influence. The case against Charlotte Bryant [51] who poisoned Frederick her husband with arsenic, may have been coloured by expectations that women should not be promiscuous. It has been suggested that Florence Maybrick [21] convicted of poisoning her husband with arsenic may have been treated unfairly before and during her trial in part because she was a woman.

'Strain theory' suggests that crime arises from tensions. They may be between society's cultural goals and structural social limitations relating to financial aspirations (Merton 1938) or to strivings for status and self-reliance (Agnew 2001). This may partly explain some poison killings.

Conclusion

As Rowland (1960) suggests, poisoners may show great ruthlessness especially when they administer the substance knowing and witnessing its effects on the victim. Of the traits suggested by Trestrail (2007) those of being: cunning, able to design and plan in detail, and (mentally and physically) non-confrontational, seem fitting.

Trestrail's (2007) typology categorising poisoners according to the extent of their planning, and the specificity of their victims, fits some poisoning cases. Quick planning and a specific victim appears to describe Susan Barber's [71] killing if her husband with Paraquat soon after he had beaten her and her lover, having found them in flagrante delicto. Quick planning and random victim seems to describe farmer Daniel Bondeson's [83] poisoning of a fellow church worshiper against whom he had no direct grudge only a generalised distaste of the church congregation. Slow planning and at least quasi random victim applies to the poisoning by Sadamichi Hirasawa [56] of bank employees so that he could rob the bank, given that he had no specific person in mind when he planned the poisoning. Similarly nurse Victorino Chua [98] carefully planned her injecting of insulin into saline bags and ampules that were later unwittingly used by other nurses.

Probably the most widely recognised and the most typical of the combinations is that of a slow planning and a specific victim. Motives relating to: money, elimination of someone or something blocking a desired goal, jealousy, revenge and political motives in one grouping as well as in another grouping sadism; belief in one's mental superiority; the desire to tamper; boredom-related challenge to law enforcement—all these fit some scenarios of poisoning.

The marked over representation of male offenders that typifies general homicides is not reflected in figures for poisoning homicides where male predominance is much less. If in the past female poisoning was more prevalent than male, it may be because of barriers to divorce for women in unhappy marriages and the opportunity afforded to women poisoners by their traditional roles in caring, and in preparing food. Peak offender ages for general and poison homicide appear similar being from late teens to early 30s. Figures allowing race comparison between homicide in general and poison homicide do not appear to be available. But for poison killings, offender and victim are usually of the same race. Illustrative cases indicate that medical professionals and others with legitimate access to poisons are over represented among occupations for poisoners. Those working in domestic service or in hospitality occupations also have access to food and drink being served but are less predominant than medical related poisoners.

Simultaneous poisoning makes it difficult for the perpetrator to avoid detection and the killer may: have not intended to kill; have meant to kill one person not many, have planned to disposed of the bodies, or may have no connection with the victims. Explanations of motives of general serial homicide such as thirsting for power and control through using force are less convincing with poison homicide where such force is absent. Also, whereas serial killing typically alerts the community, serial poisoning especially in a medical context can go undetected for decades. Offender profiling which can assist the investigation of non-poisoning killers (including serial killers) is unavailable with poisoners including serial poisoners where no one is aware that murders have occurred. Regarding team poisoning, sub cultural theories of mutually supported mitigation of the crime which relate to general homicide may apply. The poisoner's choice of acute or chronic poisoning is likely to reflect the circumstances of the homicide for example externally imposed time constraints, or a wish to have death appear to be from a wasting illness.

Theories that can inform understanding of poisoning generally include a theory of moral reasoning (Kohlberg 1978); rational choice theory (Clarke 1992); feminism and a 'gendered' view of crime (e.g., Gelsthorpe and Morris 1982); and 'strain theory' (Merton 1938; Agnew 2001).

Suggested Activities

From the glossary, identify several poisoners with different occupations. Consider the extent if any of the influence that occupation may have had on the poison used.

Key Texts

Daniszewska (2017) *Serial Homicide: Profiling of Victims and Offenders for Policing* New York, Springer

A thoughtful overview.

Dobrin (2016) *Homicide Data Sources: An Interdisciplinary Overview for Researchers* New, York, Springer

A useful guide to interpreting homicide data.

References

Agnew, R. (2001). Strain theory. In E. McLaughlin, & J. Muncie (Eds.), *The sage dictionary of criminology*. London: Sage.

Alison, L. (Ed.). (2005). *Forensic Psychologist's Casebook: Psychological Profiling and Criminal Investigation*. Devon, UK and Portland OR: Willan.

Becker, H. (1963). *Outsiders*. New York: Free Press.

Behavioural Analysis Unit. (2005). *Serial murders: Multi-disciplinary perspectives for investigators*. National Center for the Analysis of Violent Crime.

Brookman, F. (2005). *Understanding homicide*. London and Los Angeles: Sage.

Clarke, R. V. (Ed.). (1992). *Situational crime prevention: Successful case studies*. New York: Harrow and Heston.

Cohen, A. (1957). *Delinquent Boys*. Glencoe: Free Press.

Daniszewska, A. (2017). *Serial homicide: Profiling of victims and offenders for policing*. New York: Springer.

Dobrin, A. (2016). *Homicide data sources: An interdisciplinary overview for researchers (Springer briefs in criminology)*. New York: Springer.

Farrell, M. (1993). What's your poison?. *Solicitors Journal*, March 19 1993.

Farrell, M. (1994). Adelaide bartlett and the pimlico mystery. *British Medical Journal, 6970*(308), 1720–1723.

Federal Bureau of Investigation. (2015a). United States, 2014 Uniform Crime Reports Homicide Data 'Expanded Homicide Data, Table 3, Murder Offenders by Age, Sex, Race and Ethnicity, 2014' Washington DC, Federal Bureau of Investigation (https://ucr.fbi.gov/crime-in-the-u.s/2014/crime-in-the-u.s.-2014/offenses-known-to-law-enforcement/expanded-homicide)

Fox, J. A., & Levin, J. (2011). *Extreme killing: Understanding serial and mass murder*. Thousand Oaks: Sage.

Gelsthorpe, L., & Morriss, A. (1982). Feminism and criminology in Britain. *British Journal of Criminology, 28*.

Holmes, R. M., & Holmes, S. T. (2001). (2nd. ed.). *Murder in America*. London: Sage.

Holmes, R. M., & Holmes, S. T. (2010). (3rd ed.). *Serial murder*. London: Sage.

Hough, R. M., & McCorkle, K. D. (2017). *American homicide*. Thousand Oaks: Sage.

Jeffrey, C. R. (1965). Criminal behaviour and learning theory. *Journal of Criminal Law, Criminology and Police Science, 56*, 294–300.

Kelleher, M. D., & Kelleher, C. L. (1998). *Murder Most Rare: The Female Serial Killer*. Westport. CT: Praeger.

Kinnell, H. G. (2000). Serial homicide by doctors: Shipman in perspective. *British Medical Journal, 321*, 1594–1597.

Kohlberg, L. (1978). Revisions in the theory and practice of mental development. In W. Damon (Ed.), *New directions in child development: Moral development*. San Francisco: Jessey-Bass.

Laub, J., & Sampson, R. (2003). *Shared beginnings divergent lives: Delinquent boys to age 70*. Cambridge: Harvard University Press.

Lester, D. (1995). *Serial killers: The insatiable passion*. Philadelphia: Charles Press.

Merton, R. K. (1938). Social structure and anomie. *American Sociological Review, 3*, 672–682.

Mitchell, E. W. (1997). *The aetiology of serial murder towards an integrated model*. Unpublished M. Phil. Thesis.

Phillips & Bowling. (2012). 'Ethnicities, racism, crime and criminal justice' (5th ed). *The Oxford handbook of criminology oxford*. Oxford University Press, pp. 370–397.

Rappaport, R. G. (1988). The serial and mass murderer: Patterns, differentiation, pathology. *American Journal of Forensic Psychiatry, 9*, 38–48.

Ressler, R., Burgess, A., & Douglas, J. (1988). *Sexual homicide: Patterns and motives*. New York: Lexington.

Rowland, J. (1960). *Poisoner in the dock: Twelve studies of poisoning*. London: Arco.

Simpson, K. (1978). *Forty years of murder*. London: Harper Collins.

Trestrail, J. H. (2007). (2nd ed.). *Criminal poisoning: Investigational guide for law enforcement, toxicologists, forensic scientists and attorneys*. Totowa, NJ: Humana Press.

Watson, K. (2004). *Poisoned lives: English poisoners and their victims*. New York: Hambledon and London.

Westveer, A. E., Jarvis, J. P., & Jensen, C. J. (2004). *Homicidal poisoning—The silent offence. FBI Law Enforcement Bill.* August 2004, pp. 1–8.

Westveer, A. E., Trestrail, J. H., & Pinizotto, J. (1996). Homicidal poisonings in the United States—An analysis of the Uniform Crime Reports from 1980 through 1989. *American Journal of Forensic Medicine and Pathology, 17*(4), 282–288.

Chapter 8
Victims of Poisoning

Introduction

If insights can be gained from identifying characteristics of poisoners, the same applies to victims. Gender, age, race, occupation/social background and relationships between perpetrator and victim, and the location of the crime all justify examination. Not only these factors, but their interrelationships can be illuminating. Detailed information on the victim is also useful.

US Homicide Statistics

In the US, 2014 Uniform Crime Reports (UCR) homicide data provides information including the gender, age and race of victims of homicide. For example, see the 'Expanded Homicide Data, Table 2, Murder Victims by Age, Sex, Race and Ethnicity, 2014' (Federal Bureau of Investigation 2015). Figures from this database are provided in several sections later in this chapter to set the context for discussing poison homicide.

US Poison Homicide Statistics

An epidemiological study of poisonings in the US by Westveer et al. (1996) examined UCR data kept by the Department of Justice from 1980 to 1989. The UCR report submitted annually by police agencies across the US, provides

M. Farrell, *Criminology of Homicidal Poisoning*,
DOI 10.1007/978-3-319-59117-9_8

victim and offender information for various crimes. It includes the month, year and state; victim and offender information (gender, age, race), classification of the poisonous agent (drug, non-drug, fume), relationship between offender and victim, and a classification of motive. In the analysis period 202, 785 homicides were reported of which 292 involved a single offender poisoning a single victim, representing 14 poison cases per 10,000 homicides. Of the whole population, per million people poisoning averaged 1.47 per year. Westveer et al. (2004) repeated the earlier study, analysing data for 1990–1999 and showing similar findings, although with an increase in poisonings of 29% over the value in the earlier study.

Shepherd and Ferslew (2009) looked at US homicidal poisoning deaths, interrogating the National Mortality Statistics database for the years 1999–2005. Counts and rates were obtained for subgroupings by using demographic data and *ICD-10* codes (a World Health Organisation classification of diseases). In all, 523 homicidal poisoning deaths were identified. Overall homicidal poisoning death rate between 1999 and 2005 was low at 0.26/million/year. Medications were the most common poison. Rates were significantly higher than average for the country in the West of the US and lower in the Northeast.

While such figures help to provide a broad context, it is the more detailed comparisons of general homicide and poison homicide regarding gender, age and race and occupation/social background that is more informative as we shall see.

Gender of Victim: Statistics

Homicide in General

In the US, 2014 UCR homicide data indicates that the rounded percent distribution for males was 77.3% and for females was 22.4% (for 0.3% of victims the gender was not known) (Federal Bureau of Investigation 2015).

Poison Homicide

Examining homicidal poisoning deaths in the US, 1999–2005 indicates that males were significantly more likely to be victims than females (Shepherd and Ferslew 2009). However, analysis of the 1980–1989 UCR data on poisoning homicides (Westveer et al. 1996) showed that the number of male and female victims was about equal. If the victim was female, the offender was usually male; whereas if the victim was male, the offender was equally likely to be male or female.

Gender of Victim: Illustrative Poisoning Cases

Male-on-Male Poisoning

In the past and into the present time, men killing men has constituted the majority of criminal homicides. While confrontational homicide using a firearm, knife or bludgeon is the most common form of motivation and medium, premeditated acts can lead to poison being used as the choice weapon (Hough and McCorkle 2017, private communication). Male-on-male homicides in general are characterised by violent confrontation or revenge. However, male-on-male poisonings are typically not violently confrontational, but are more considered.

Examples of male on male poisoning include a rival being murdered. Ryan Furlough [86] killed his friend Benjamin Vassilev with cyanide out of jealousy. Steven Roy Harper [69] used *N*-Nitrosodimethylamine to poison Duane Johnson the husband of Sandra Johnson, Harper's former girlfriend (and their 11-month-old son Chad) out of jealousy. From professional rather than romantic rivalry, Adolph Hofrichter [36] killed fellow officer Captain Richard Mader with potassium cyanide capsules. Where male doctors or nurses kill their patients these may be male or female.

Male–on-male poisoning can be motivated by greed. Reginald Hinks [48] gassed James Pullen, his father-in-law, with carbon monoxide (in coal gas) for financial gain. Dr. George Lamson [17] poisoned his brother-in-law Percy John with aconite for similar reasons. In depression-hit New York, a group of men including Dan Keisberg [47] conspired to poison (with carbon monoxide coal gas) down-and-out Mike Malloy, whose life they had insured.

Male-on-Female Poisoning

Poison femicide often involves the perpetrator poisoning a spouse or lover. Wife killers include Carlyle Harris [24] (using morphine), Paul Marshall Curry [95] (nicotine injection), Eugène Chantrelle [16] (opium), and Arthur Deveureux [31] (morphine). Medical poisoners (and those in related professions) who killed their wives used various poisons and drugs, informed by their professional knowledge. These included succinylcholine chloride (Nurse Charles Higgs) [90], morphine (Dr. Robert Buchanan) [25], arsenic (Dr. Philip Cross) [20], aconite and antimony (Dr. Edward Pritchard)v [12] and cyanide (Dr. Robert Ferrante) [97]. Poisoners who killed lovers include Walter Horsford [27] and George Chapman [29]. Roger and David Cooper [99] chloroformed and killed Roger Cooper's lover Sameena Imam. Among other cases is that of Reverend Frank Sipple [54] who used a cyanide capsule to murder his daughter. Israel Lipski [19] used nitric acid to poison Miriam Angel a fellow resident in a lodging house. George Trepal [77] killed his neighbour

Peggy Carr with thallium following a dispute. Frederick Seddon [37] killed his lodger Eliza Barrow with arsenic.

It is unclear how many of these poisonings were influenced by a perpetrator's desire to exert control, as is the case with some non-poisoning femicides, which may emerge from a history of domestic abuse. Certainly, a spouse or lover who is being poisoned cannot subsequently adapt to control because they are typically unaware that they are being killed. However, chronic poisoners may be motivated by the desire to control, having power over the victim's protracted suffering. In the typology of Fox and Levin (2011) mentioned in the earlier chapter on poisoners, recall that the most common type is thought to be the serial killer thirsting for power and control who uses force (Ibid. pp. 23–26). Along these lines, Dr. Harold Shipman [81] may have been driven by feelings of power achieved through serial poisoning.

Female on Male Poisoning

When women kill, the victim is often a spouse. Among reasons for this is likely the opportunity to administer poison to someone with whom one is in close daily contact, for example perhaps preparing and/or serving their food. Among spouse killers are Stella Nickell [75] (cyanide), Susan Barber [71] (Paraquat), Mary Wilson [64] (phosphorus), Ethel Major [49] (strychnine), Angelina Rodriguez [84] (ethylene glycol-based antifreeze), and Kristin Rossum [82] (fentanyl). Other examples are Charlotte Bryant [51], Marie Hilley [70], Maria Groesbeek [67], Edith Carew [26] and Marie Lafarge [4] who all used arsenic in different forms. Blanche Moore [78] used arsenic to kill her boyfriend Raymond Reid. An example of a non-spouse female on male poisoning is Amy Archer-Gilligan's [41] killing of Franklin Andrews, a former resident of her Connecticut Nursing Home.

Female-on-Female Poisoning

Jealousy, either romantic or professional can be a motive in female-on-female poisoning. Hélèna Jégado [7] in France administered arsenic in food and drink to Perotte Mace a fellow hotel worker; and later to Rose Tessier and Rosalie Sarrazin (both fellow domestic servants) out of professional jealousy. Cordelia Botkin [28] sent arsenic in chocolates by post to her lover's estranged wife, Mary Dunning, killing both her and Mary's sister Ida Deane. In Indonesia, Jessica Wongso [100] jealously poisoned her former friend Wayan Salihin with cyanide-laced coffee.

Financial gain is another motive. Housekeeper, Louisa Merrifield [58] administered rat poison containing phosphorus to her employer Sarah Anne Ricketts. Dorothea Waddingham [50] a nursing home manager gave overdoses of morphine tablets to kill Louisa Baguley and her daughter Ada Baguley. K.D. Kempanna [94] in India killed six women temple worshipers using cyanide. Greed was behind all these killings.

Age of Victim: Statistics

Homicide in General

In the US 2014, UCR data (released 2015) indicates that the age bands with the highest numbers and proportions of victims are those between 20 and 39 years and especially 20–24 years (Federal Bureau of Investigation 2015). Despite natural and sometimes justified worries of parents that their child might be harmed by strangers, Brookman (2005) observes that child homicide victims are most likely to be killed by their parents and very few children are killed by someone unknown to them (Ibid. p. 187).

Poison Homicide

Analysis of the 1980–1989 UCR data for poison homicide (Westveer et al. 1996) showed that the highest number of victims was aged 25–29 years; and that the highest number of offenders was aged 20–34 years. The age range of victims was from a single instance of a baby of less than 1 week old to 13 victims of 75 years or older. Shepherd and Ferslew (2009) in their study of US homicidal poisoning deaths 1999–2005 found that killing was more likely at extremes of age. Rates were 2.05/million in children younger than 1 year and 0.56/million at ages 85 years or older.

Age of Victim: Illustrative Poisoning Cases

Child victims may be poisoned by their own parents (or step parents). John Armstrong [62] murdered his five month old son Terence with Seconal sodium. Steven Roy Harper [69] used *N*-Nitrosodimethylamine to poison Duane Johnson the husband of Sandra Johnson (Harper's former girlfriend) and their 11 month old son Chad. Arthur Deveureux [31] used morphine to kill his two year old twin sons (and his wife). Timothy O'Bryan was eight years old when his father Ronald Clark O'Bryan [73] killed him with potassium cyanide. Teresa Miriam Conroy [57] poisoned her 13 year old son with carbon-monoxide gas and methylphenobarbitone and was judged to be guilty but insane.

Where a child is the victim it may be maintained that the perpetrator is experiencing *factitious disorder imposed on another* (American Psychiatric Association 2013, pp. 324–327). This form of abuse, usually of a child, involves a parent (typically the child's biological mother) or carer causing or inventing symptoms of illness in the child in order to attract admiration or sympathy for themselves. The perpetrator may harm the victim to sustain the supposed illness. Genene Jones [74] used succinylcholine to kill 15-month-old Chelsea McClellan and heparin to poison another child Rolando Santos. A pediatric nurse, she endangered the lives of the children in her care then sought adulation by 'saving' them. Lacey Spears [96] appeared to be a devoted mother whose son Garnett-Paul was often ill, while in reality she was poisoning the child with salt, and finally administered a lethal dose.

In Victorian England where domestic servants and nursemaids were common there were sometimes poisonings of employer's children (Watson 2004, p. 131). But generally where a child is poisoned by someone other than their parents, the circumstances are unusual as when dentist Dr. Etienne Deschamps [23] chloroformed to death 12-year-old Juliette Deitsh, whom he had been sexually abusing when he feared this would be revealed.

Also vulnerable are victims of advanced age when death might be expected. Many of the 250 victims of serial poisoner Dr. Harold Shipman [81] were elderly, the oldest being 93–year-old Anne Cooper. Yukiko Shimoyama poisoned with vecuronium bromide by the nurse Daisuke Mori [89] at a clinic in Japan, was 89 years old. One of the nursing home patients poisoned by Dorothea Waddingham [50] for financial gain was 89-year-old Louisa Baguley. Sarah Anne Ricketts was 79 years old when poisoned with rat poison containing phosphorus by her housekeeper and companion Louisa Merrifield [58]. In Portland, Maine, farmer Daniel Bondeson [83] killed Walter Morrill aged 78 a fellow church worshiper, with arsenic administered in the after service coffee. Victims of Mary Wilson [64] through phosphorus poisoning were her second husband Oliver Leonard aged 75, and her third husband Ernest Wilson aged 76. Reginald Hinks [48] murdered his 74-year-old father-in-law with carbon monoxide.

Race of Victim: Statistics

Homicide in General

Statistics involving race or ethnicity involve classifications that are inconsistent and sometimes overlapping (Phillips and Bowling 2012, p. 372). Using a basic categorisation, US 2014 data (released 2015) indicates that of murder victims for whom race was known, the rounded percent distribution was, 51.0% black, 45.1% white, and 2.6% other races. (Race was unknown for 1.3% victims) (Federal Bureau of Investigation 2015).

Poison Homicide

The 1980–1989 UCR data for poison homicide (Westveer, Trestrail and Pinizotto, 1996) indicated that victim and offender were usually of the same race. Victims were most often white. If the victim was white, the offender was usually male; while if the victim was black, the offender could equally be male or female. Twice as many black victims were male than female. There were equal numbers of white female and white male victims. Finally, for black or white offenders, there were twice as many males as females.

Shepherd and Ferslew (2009) analysing US homicidal poisoning deaths 1999–2005, found that rates varied by race and were more common among Blacks (0.43/million). The greatest rate was observed in Black infants (5.3/million). Given the very broad categorisation of simply, 'black' and 'white' it is unclear what if any conclusions can be made from these figures.

Race of Victim: Illustrative Poisoning Cases

As previously noted, the racial identity of the victim is generally the same as that of the perpetrator. More broadly, this intra-racial pattern is true of almost all crimes. Spouse murders and murders of relatives are common in poisonings, and as these relationships tend to be within the same racial groups, so are killings. In 2015, Lakvir Singh [93] a Sikh living in London, was convicted of killing her Sikh lover Lakhvinder Cheema with aconite acquired on a visit to India. In China, Wei Entan [87] killed his lover's child and one of the child's classmates, with rat poison in 2003, the perpetrator and the victims all being Chinese. The six women temple worshipers killed by K.D. Kempanna [94] with cyanide between 1997 and 2007 around temples in the state of Karnataka, appear to have all been Indian devotees.

An example of poisoning where the perpetrator and victim have different racial origins is that of Roger and David Cooper [99], both Caucasian, poisoning with chloroform, Roger Cooper's lover Sameena Imam, who was of Indian origin. In other examples, where the perpetrator is a serial poisoner and where the victims are patients in a hospital or in the community, depending on the ethnic composition of the patient group there is the possibility of killings across racial groupings.

Occupation/Social Class of Victim: Illustrative Poisoning Cases

Social class can be categorised by a range of indicators such as income, type of housing and occupation. All else being equal, occupation and social class of a victim of poisoning can be expected, to be similar to that of the poisoner. This is because a poisoner tends to be known sometimes intimately to the victim, which provides the opportunity for poison to be secretly administered in food or drink or in some other way. Where the victim is the spouse of a poisoner, they are usually of similar social status.

Hippolyte Ballet killed by Dr. Edme Castaing [3] with morphine acetate powder, was the doctor's conspirator in an earlier fraud. Rosalie Sarrazin poisoned by Hélèna Jégado [7] was a fellow servant girl. John Cooke, administered strychnine by Dr. William Palmer [8], was the physician's gambling companion. Miriam Angel killed by Israel Lipski [19] with nitric acid, was a resident in the same lodging house. Captain Richard Mader was killed out of jealousy by Adolph Hofrichter [36], a fellow officer, who used potassium cyanide capsules, sent through the post. Louis Pernotte was an insurance agent while Henri Girrard [42] his killer was an insurance swindler.

Where there are wide differences in social status, this may be owing to a professional or business relationship. Frau Glaser, Judge Grohmann and Frau Gebhardt, the victims of arsenic poisoner Anna Zwanziger [2] reflected her own status as housekeeper, as they were either her direct employers or their spouses. Sarah Anne Ricketts was the victim of Louisa Merrifield [58] her house keeper who administered to her rat poison containing phosphorus. Secretaries June Malins and Betty Grant were poisoned by Arthur Ford [60], general manager of a manufacturing chemist using cantharides. Bob Egle and Fred Biggs were murdered by their poison obsessed work colleague Graham Young [68], using thallium. More unusually, landlord and landlady Richard and Elizabeth Beck died from prussic acid intended for their tenant by Richard Brinkley [33]. Helen Donworth, Matilda Clover, Emma Showell and Alice Marsh, were prostitutes killed by Dr. Neill Cream [22] with strychnine. Mike Malloy a down and out alcoholic in depression-hit New York, was chosen for murder after a group of men including Dan Keisberg [47] had insured his life. The gang then killed him using carbon monoxide gas.

Offender–Victim Relationship: Statistics

Homicide in General

In male-on-male homicides often the participants are acquaintances (30%) or strangers (20%) after which come friends (10%) and family members (7%) (Brookman 2005, p. 122). A different picture emerges for femicide, in which over a half of women victims are killed by their current or former boyfriend, husband or lover (intimate femicide). Less than 10% are killed by a stranger (Ibid. p. 141). Also, when women kill, it tends to be intimate partners or ex-partners and family members (their children) (Ibid. pp. 162–163).

Poison Homicide

Watson (2004) analysing poison cases from Assizes Records 1750–1914 in England and Wales found that of accused poisoners, 60% targeted members of their immediate family. If one adds to these poisoning carried out by servants (who were members of the family by law and custom) and including nurses and nursemaids who lived in the home, the figure rises to 70% (Ibid. p. 48 and p. 45 Table 4). Lovers, neighbours, colleagues and friends made up a further 13%. Another group were medical attendants and 'professional' abortionists. Other than these, only 10% of identified poisoners had a distant relationship with their victims (Ibid. p. 48).

The 1980–1989 UCR data (Westveer et al. 1996) suggested that many victims did not have a relationship with the offender's family (despite the expectation that most homicidal poisonings would involve a domestic environment).

Offender–Victim Relationship: Illustrative Poison Cases

Illustrative cases indicate the range of relationships pertaining in poison cases. These include: family relationships (spouse/partner, parent/child, other relatives, housekeeper, and lodger as de facto family member), lover and rival in love, patient-medic and other relationships. As noted above, there are also cases where the victim was a stranger to the perpetrator.

Actual and de Facto Family Relationships

Numerous wives and husbands have poisoned their spouses as illustrated earlier in this chapter and in the glossary which outlines many other examples. Instances where a parent has poisoned their child include the Reverend Frank Sipple [54], a US Pastor who used a cyanide capsule to kill his 18-year-old daughter Dorothy Ann Sipple at the family home Grand Rapids, Michigan. Ronald Clark O'Bryan [73] used potassium cyanide administered in candy to kill Timothy his 8-year-old son to gain from life insurance. Teresa Miriam Conroy [57] was judged insane after killing her 13-year-old son, at their home in London with carbon monoxide gas and methylphenobarbitone. In England, John Armstrong [62], a sick berth attendant at a naval hospital, poisoned his 5-month-old-son with Seconal sodium in capsules. Where perpetrators kill someone else's child the motive is likely to be revenge or jealousy. This was evident with Steven Roy Harper [69] who killed a former girlfriend's 11-month-old-baby out of jealousy; and Wei Entan [87] who, out of revenge that his married lover was ending their affair, poisoned her son and daughter.

Jane Cowan, murdered by Dr. Edward Pritchard [12] with aconite (and antimony) was the physician's, mother-in-law. Percy John, killed by aconite administered by Dr. George Lamson [17] was the medic's brother-in-law. Alice Pearson poisoned with strychnine by Sarah Anne Pearson and Agnes Black (born Pearson) [30], was Agnes' mother and Sarah's mother-in-law. Hannah and John Peck killed by Arthur Waite [40], using diphtheria and tuberculosis germs were his in-laws. James Pullen was killed by Reginald Hinks [48], his son-in-law, using carbon monoxide.

Housekeepers are necessarily conversant with family routines. Among these is Anna Zwanziger [2] in Germany who administered arsenic in food and drink to several of her employers; and Louisa Merrifield [58] who killed her employer Sarah Anne Ricketts with phosphorus-based rat poison. Where there is a lodger in a family home, both lodger and family can become familiar with each other's habits and circumstances so that if murder is contemplated, poisoning might be considered. In London, Catherine Wilson [64] was a housekeeper and live-in nurse, but it appears that when she poisoned Maria Soames, with colchicum, she was more of a lodger in the house. Frederick Seddon [37] a London-based insurance superintendent, poisoned his lodger Eliza Barrow for financial gain. In Vienna, Austria, Martha Marek [53] used thallium to kill a lodger Frau Kittenberger (among others). Where the setting is a lodging house where there can be many residents again one person may get insights into the daily routines of others. Israel Lipski [19] an umbrella stick maker may have known when his victim was likely to be alone when he forcefully administered nitric acid to Miriam Angel a married fellow resident in their boarding house. In most of these cases, the intimacy of the family circle allows access to the food and drink consumed by the victim, and knowledge of their habits and preferences that can facilitate poisoning.

Lovers and Rivals

Perhaps inevitably, passion including jealousy is a feature of many poisonings involving lovers and rivals. Sarah Hadler an unwanted mistress who had borne two children by Quaker John Tawell [5] met her death when Tawell administered prussic acid to her, because he was worried that his wife would discover the relationship. Seraphine de Pawr killed with digitalis by Dr. Edmund de la Pommerais [11] was his mistress. Maud Marsh died of antimony poison administered by George Chapman [29] her lover. Avis Linnell, killed with potassium cyanide by Reverend Clarence Richeson [38], had been his lover and the pastor was planning to marry someone else. Sameena Imam was killed using chloroform by her lover Roger Cooper and his brother [99]. Alfred Jones was poisoned by Jean Pierre Vaquier [45] who was the lover of Jones's wife Mabe. Cordelia Botkin [28] killed Mary Dunning the wife of her lover with arsenic impregnated chocolates.

Patient-Medic

At least four patients were killed with arsenic by Dr. Michael Swango [80]. It is estimated that 250 patients were killed by Dr. Harold Shipman [81] using mainly morphine-based drugs. Nurse poisoners who killed their patients include: Orville Lynn Majors [79] (using potassium chloride), Marie Jeanneret [13] (belladonna), Dorothea Waddingham [50] (morphine) and Victorino Chua [98] (insulin). Nursing home manager Amy Archer-Gilligan [41] killed her patients with arsenic; Norwegian Arnfinn Nessett [72] used succinylcholine chloride, and Donald Harvey [76] used cyanide as well as other poisons and other methods. Pediatric nurse Genene Jones [74] poisoned children including a 15-month-old baby under her medical care.

Other Relationships

Work relationships and roles, and friendships or former friendships can bring poisoners within the close orbit of their victims. Such relationships can provide fertile ground for intense emotions that can lead to violence including murder. June Malins and Betty Grant poisoned with cantharides by Arthur Ford [60] were secretaries in the office that he managed. Bob Egle and Fred Biggs, poisoned by Graham Young [68] with thallium, were his work colleagues. Benjamin Vassilev was killed by his onetime friend Ryan Furlough [86] using cyanide. Annie Hamann was inadvertently killed by her friend Christa Lehman [59] using E605 when the poisoner was planning to kill Karl Lehman her husband, and Valentin Lehman her father-in-law (and did so).

Stranger

Given the often intimate nature of poisoning, it is unusual that a victim is a complete stranger to a homicidal poisoner. The poisoner may feign a position of trust to entrap victims. Over a period of several years in war-torn France some 24 people were killed Dr. Marcel Petiot [55] using cyanide. All came to him with the promise of escape. In Japan, several members of bank staff were given cyanide pellets by Sadamichi Hirasawa [56], who posed as an official and convinced them that they were taking an immunisation. Product tampering is sometimes used to cover a murder by spreading suspicion. Bank manager Susan Snow, was randomly killed with cyanide when Stella Nickell [75] who had murdered her husband Bruce with the poison tampered with local shop products to try to conceal her crime.

A stranger can be killed inadvertently where a perpetrator plans to murder another person but the plan backfires. Richard and Elizabeth Beck died from consuming a drink laced with prussic acid left on a table by Richard Brinkley [33] who intended it for a potential witness to forgery Reginald Parker.

Location of Homicide: Statistics

Homicide in General

For homicide in general the killing is patterned in both space and time. Regarding location, a study analysed homicides observed in three police forces in England and Wales 1994–1996 (Brookman 2000). This study indicated that the most common venue was a house (52%) followed by street (16%), 'open space' (15%) and 'public house/club (9%). The 'house' could be that of the offender, the victim, or a dwelling shared by both, or the home of a friend—most common was the house of a victim or one shared by both offender and victim (Ibid.). Street, open space and public house setting can involve a deadly mix of offence given and taken, alcohol and public setting and intense emotions or an argument. This leaves the percentage of home-based killings with the realm of intimate partner homicide, domestic violence and the murder of loved ones or family (Hough and McCorkle 2017, personal communication).

Poison Homicide

Ready statistics regarding the physical location of most homicides by poison are hard to come by. Part of the reason for this, at least in the US, stems from the various reporting mechanisms. Each of some 18,000 separate law enforcement agencies reports certain aspects of homicide cases to the state level. Each state then aggregates such data to submit to the FBI for inclusion in the annual UCR. State level health agencies and bureaus of vital statistics also report various data regarding recorded death cases of all sorts. The Centers for Disease Control (CDC) of the US government also compiles deaths identified as homicide in yet another aggregate report (Hough and McCorkle 2017). However illustrative poison cases can shed some light on possible locations.

Location of the Homicide: Illustrative Poison Cases

A rural location can involve poisons available in the locality including plant poisons, fertilizers, and poisons used to dispatch vermin. An urban setting might involve poisons being acquired from a factory or stolen from a large store. Often reflecting the domestic nature of many homicidal poisonings, the place of the killing is the home. Toxicologist Kristin Rossum [82] poisoned her husband with fentanyl at their La Jollia residence having telephoned his office to say that he would not be coming into work that day.

Other venues include a place where medicines are stored and administered such as a nursing home, hospital, or doctor's surgery. Dr. Harold Shipman [81] although he killed most of his patients at their respective homes also occasionally killed in his surgery. Poison has also been administered in more public places. Jessica Wongso [100] poisoned her friend Wayan Salihin in a busy cafe in Jakarta, Indonesia by lacing her coffee with cyanide.

Settings other than the place where the deceased died may be important. As Trestrail (2007) points out these include potentially different places where the poison was procured, prepared, administered, and discarded (Ibid. p. 70). Procurement may have been through the Internet, from a legitimate supply (as with many medical murders), or from a source obtained illegally, for example through stealing. John Armstrong [62] probably stole the Seconal sodium with which he killed his baby son from the naval hospital where he worked. Roger Cooper [99] purchased chloroform through e-bay and with his brother David, used it to kill Roger Cooper's lover Sameena Imam.

A poison-requiring preparation may have been made ready in a different place to where it was administered. Count Hippolyte de Bocarmé [6] distilled nicotine in a secluded part of his home and administered it (forcibly) to his brother-in-law Gustave Fougnies in the dining room.

Where the action of a poison is rapid, then the venue where the poison was administered may be the same one as that where death took place. This was so when Jean Pierre Vaquier [45] killed Alfred Jones, proprietor of the Blue Anchor Hotel, England with strychnine added to the landlord's health salts. Sometimes, the place of administering the poison and the venue where the victim dies are distant. Bob Egle and Fred Biggs did not die at work where he was poisoned at work by Graham Young [68] because the thallium that he used acts over a prolonged period of time. The place where the poison is disposed of may be close to where the death took place as with the killing of Elizabeth Barlow with insulin injection, where the syringes were found adjacent to the bathroom where Kenneth Barlow [63] her husband committed the crime. Alternatively, attempts may be made to destroy the poison as with Charlotte Bryant [51], who tried to incinerate the tin of arsenical weed killer that she had used to poison her husband Frederick.

Interaction of Characteristics, Relationship and Location

Information on gender, age, race and occupation/social class, offender–victim relationship and location of homicide can be illuminating. Further insight can be gain by looking at combinations of these factors. Also important is the interplay of factors relevant to understanding perpetrator-victim interactions and other relationships.

In India, K.D. Kempanna [94] chose other women temple worshipers as victims. Meeting them on several occasions, she ensured that they had money or valuables and gained their trust. For the killings, she chose a remote temple suggested by her so that there would be no witnesses to the violent reaction that cyanide has on victims. Gender, apparent-shared interests, location and social standing all interact to provide the back cloth of the killings.

It appears that age played a part when Lakvir Singh [93] killed her lover Lakhvinder 'Lucky' Cheema with aconite. When in October 2008 after a 16-year secret affair, Cheema wanted to end their relationship, Lakvir Singh was 45, and Cheema's new fiancé Gurjeet Choongh was aged 21. Probably the rage and jealousy that Singh expressed prior to the killing was fuelled by this age discrepancy as well as the obvious unfairness to her mind of what was transpiring. Cheema's house was one of the few locations, where Singh could be sure that the pair would be together and would eat the same food. As she no longer had the easy access to the house that she had previously enjoyed, she had to try to surreptitiously introduce the poison into the food that they would eat that night.

Farmer Daniel Bondeson's [83] crimes were part of the fabric of the Lutheran Church that he attended and where there had been internal disputes. His generalised grievance to the whole congregation explains why the arsenic was introduced to the coffee supply for everyone rather than directed at a particular person. Walter Morrill happened to be the one who died although others also became ill. The locality of the farming community gave access to arsenic in old farm chemical products.

When Jessica Wongso [100] killed her friend with cyanide-laced coffee in a shopping mall café in Jakarta, Indonesia, their similar age and the fact that they had studied together and become friends becomes part of the background. It informs Jessica Wongso's jealousy towards Wayan Salihin who was clearly more successful and had recently been happily married. A public setting may have been chosen to paradoxically provide 'cover' for the poisoning as it provided inadvertent witnesses. Wongso seems to have planned sufficiently to place items on a table to block the view of CCTV cameras as she tampered with her friend's drink.

Gathering Detailed Information on the Victim

Victim's Recent Contacts

As well as broad features of victims in general, specific information about a victim in particular will be gathered by investigators. This is likely to include working out the victim's recent movements and contacts. From witnesses, including any doctor who treated the victim in life, the state of health of the victim can be established. They may have been in previously good health and then suddenly have become unexplainably ill.

Questions may arise. Did the victim complain of any symptoms such gastrointestinal upset? Did they experience convulsions which without other plausible explanations might suggest poisoning by strychnine for example? Did they experience local or generalised paralysis which could suggest cyanide, thallium and several other poisons? Did they fall into a coma before death, which might point to poisons such as opiates; or carbon monoxide poisoning? What did they recently eat or drink? If the deceased vomited any traces of it will need to be collected. Did the deceased recently receive any unsolicited parcels (that may have contained poison disguised in a gift)?

Victim's Routines and Preferences

Routines followed by the victim may be used by the poisoner to enable the crime. The victim may eat certain food and consume certain favourite drinks that can be exploited. A soft drink was an obvious choice for Ryan Furlough [86] who laced it with cyanide and gave it to his friend Benjamin Vassilev because they regularly consumed such drinks. A favourite food or drink (including alcohol) may be used in which to conceal the poison, given that the strength of the food's flavour is likely to mask any taste or odour from the poison. Should the victim be known to have a liking for confectionary, chocolates or similar can be offered, and have sometimes been sent through the post to kill victims.

If the victim is known to take medication at certain times, this gives the opportunity to add poison to the tonic, capsules or other medication involved. Should the victim be addicted to drugs, taking them regularly, this habit can be exploited to introduce poison. Items used solely by the victim can be doctored with poison so that only they are affected. This may be a favourite cup or flask. If the poisoner is a spouse of carer/caretaker, that can have the opportunity not only to administer the poison, put to clear away or destroy incriminating evidence, even where this involved giving poison over a lengthy period of time. If the victim is known to be in a depressed state, or if others can be convinced that the victim is in such a state, this can prepare the ground for poisoning that can be made to look like suicide.

Why Victimised?

Bringing together possible broad characteristics of victims and details about their past and most recent circumstances, can help raise the question of why they were the victim. One way of considering this is to look *from the point of view of the suspected perpetrator*, what it was about the victim and their circumstances that precipitated their killing. Studying the behaviour of people in this way to determine why they became victims has come to be known as 'victimology'. Looking at the victim in this fashion is often a mirror image of considering the possible motives of the perpetrator.

It may have been beneficial from the poisoners standpoint to get rid of the victim because they were blocking a desired goal. (This motivation is encountered in murder perpetrated by many methods). The victim may be in a relationship with the poisoner as a spouse or partner which may have cooled and become side-lined by a new relationship. This was how marriage to Walter Carew hindered his wife Edith Carew's [26] desire to be with her lover, and arsenic was her way to resolve this dilemma. South African Christian Burys blocked his wife Maria Groesbeek's [67] wish to be with her lover. In Ireland, Laura Cross thwarted Dr. Philip Cross [20] from seeing his mistress; while in Canada Sarah the wife of Dr. William King [9] similarly hindered her husband. Mary Marymont was in the way of US Master Sergeant Marcus Marymont [65] for the same reason. Where the victim is blocking desired relationships it may be in a more generalised way. Katherine Armstrong prevented her solicitor husband Herbert Armstrong [43] from general sexual freedom which he exercised in taking a holiday after killing her with arsenic. Each of the foregoing is an example of the type of goal blockage based on a romantic relationship. There are also other motivations.

A victim may provide the prospect of monetary gain. Lodger Eliza Barrow made over her wealth for an annuity for life providing the incentive (as he saw it) for Frederick Seddon [37] to kill her with arsenic. Anna Buchanan killed with morphine by her husband Dr. Robert Buchanan [25] prevented him from marrying another woman, and provided him with the prospect of financial gain.

Mary Dunning the former wife of Cordelia Botkin's [28] lover aroused the jealousy of Cordelia who killed her with arsenic impregnated chocolates. Similarly, French servant girl Rosalie Sarrazin came within the jealous prevue of Hélèna Jégado [7] who poisoned her with arsenic.

It is more difficult to see a victim from a perpetrator's point of view where they are killed for sadistic pleasure. Bob Egle and Fred Biggs, work colleagues of Graham Young [68] were killed with thallium more as an objective experiment than for any intelligible reason connected with them as people. The many patients of Norwegian nursing home manager Arnfinn Nesset [72] were killed because they were available and relatively powerless, as were the numerous patients killed by Dr. Harold Shipman [81]. In murders brought about by product tampering to cover an initial killing, the secondary victims can be quite random as when Susan Snow was killed by the cyanide introduced by Stella Nickell [75] into capsules sold in a local store to cover the poisoning of her husband Bruce.

Conclusion

For homicide in general, victims are predominantly male with over three times as many men being victims than women. Regarding homicidal poisoning either male and female victims are similar in number; or there may be more male victims, but nothing like to the same degree as for homicides generally. While male on male homicides in general are characterised by violent confrontation or revenge, male-on-male poisonings are not violently confrontational, but tend to be more considered. Femicide poisoning which often involves the killing of a spouse or lover does not appear to be explained by desire to exert control, as is the case with some non-poisoning femicides, which may emerge from a history of domestic abuse. However, chronic poisoning may be an exception to this. Female on male poisoning also tends to involve a spouse or lover. Regarding female on female poisonings, recurring motives include romantic or professional jealousy and financial gain.

Turning to age, in homicide generally, there is a peak age range for victims from about 20–40 years. For poison homicide, some research has found an age peak in the mid to late 20s, while others have shown peaks for the very young and the elderly. It is possible that there are higher levels of poisoning of elderly people than is sometimes thought given that death is often expected and therefore homicide may go undetected.

With regard to the race of victims, for homicide in general US figures show a higher proportion of black over white victims although it is unclear what the picture is for poison homicides. It appears though that poison victims and offenders are often of the same race.

The social background of poison offenders and victims tends to be similar given the usually intimate nature of poisoning for example access to the victim's food and drink.

In male on male homicides in general often the participants are acquaintances or strangers, but in femicide over a half of women victims are killed by their current or former boyfriend, husband or lover (intimate femicide). When women kill, it tends to be intimate partners or ex-partners and family members. For poison victims, again the intimate nature of poisoning suggests that there is generally a relationship between poison victim and offender. These include that of spouse, lover, relative, friend, co-worker and patient medic.

The location of many homicides in general is the home and this appears similar for poison homicides. Other poisoning venues are nursing homes and hospitals where medics are the perpetrators. Victims have also been poisoned in public places and at their place of work. With poisoning, to a greater extent than with homicides using other weapons, several locations are likely to be relevant such as where the poison was obtained, stored, administered, and discarded.

In looking at individual cases, one can begin to see how the age, gender, race and occupation of the poison victim and offender and the locations involved can interact to influence such features as role expectations and the course of events. While such interactions are not predictive, they can be informative. Knowledge of the victim's recent contacts their routines (such as medication regimes) and preferences (such as foods) and the possible reasons why they became a victim (from the point of view of a suspect) can add to the understanding of the crime. Understanding the interaction of demographic and relationship factors can aid investigators in the retroactive function of determining who committed a crime and holding them accountable through the court system.

Suggested Activities

Consider the following:

Ways in which gender, age, race and social class/occupation of perpetrator and victim (and others) might interact in particular cases that could inform understanding of what was happening and perhaps aid investigation.

Further examples in which the perpetrator's understanding of the victim's routines facilitated poisoning.

Key Texts

Doerner and Lab (6th. edition) (2012) *Victimology* New York and London, Elsevier

Although this book does not specifically consider poisoning, it usefully gives a general orientation to thinking about crime by examining victims. Early chapters on 'The Scope of Victimology' and 'Measuring Criminal Victimisation' offer an overview while Chap. 4 looks at 'Personal Victimisation' including homicide.

References

American Psychiatric Association. (2013). *Diagnostic and statistical manual of mental disorders (DSM5)*, (5th ed.). Washington, DC: APA.

Brookman, F. (2000). *Dying for control: Men, murder and sub-lethal violence in England and Wales.* Unpublished Ph.D. Thesis, Cardiff University.

Brookman, F. (2005). *Understanding homicide.* London and Los Angeles: Sage.

Federal Bureau of Investigation. (2015). United States, 2014 Uniform Crime Reports Homicide Data 'Expanded Homicide Data, Table 2, Murder Victims by Age, Sex, Race and Ethnicity, 2014' https://ucr.fbi.gov/crime-in-the-u.s/2014/crime-in-the-u.s.-2014/offenses-known-to-law-enforcement/expanded-homicide

Fox, J. A., & Levin, J. (2011). *Extreme Killing: Understanding Serial and Mass Murder.* Thousand Oaks, CA: Sage.

Hough, R. M., & McCorkle, K. D. (2017). *American homicide.* Thousand Oaks: Sage.

Phillips, C., & Bowling, B. (2012). Ethnicities, racism, crime and criminal justice. In M. Maguire, R. Morgan, & R. Reiner (Eds.), (5th ed.). *The Oxford handbook of criminology.* Oxford: Oxford University Press.

Shepherd, G., & Ferslew, B. C. (2009). Homicidal poisoning deaths in the United States 1999–2005. *Clinical Toxicology, 47*(4), 342–347.

Trestrail, J. H. (2007). *Criminal poisoning: investigational guide for law enforcement, toxicologists, forensic scientists and attorneys totowa*, (2nd ed). NJ, Humana Press.

Watson, K. (2004). *Poisoned lives: english poisoners and their victims.* New York, Hambledon and London.

Westveer, A. E., Jarvis, J. P., & Jensen, C. J. (2004). *Homicidal poisoning—The silent offence. FBI Law Enforcement Bill.* August 2004, pp. 1–8.

Westveer, A. E., Trestrail, J. H., & Pinizotto, J. (1996). Homicidal poisonings in the United States —An analysis of the Uniform Crime Reports from 1980 through 1989. *American Journal of Forensic Medicine and Pathology, 17*(4), 282–288.

Chapter 9
Detection and Its Avoidance in Poisoning Cases

Introduction

Aspects of detection that can contribute to successfully identifying the perpetrator of poisoning can all be subverted for example by the poisoner's careful planning of by errors in detection. Recall that Westveer et al. (1996) analysing 1980–1989 UCR data found that the unknown offender rate for poisoning cases was 20–30 times higher than for non-poisoning homicides.

Cause of Illness and Death and Its Distortion

Cause of Illness and Death

If a poisoner can convince others that the cause of the victim's death is natural or has an explanation not implicating the perpetrator, rigorous investigation may be circumvented. Physicians have to be alert to apparent symptoms of illness or disease being in fact indications of poisoning. Strychnine causes violent convulsions that can be mistaken for epilepsy. Symptoms of arsenic poisoning mimic heat stroke or cholera and can be mistaken by physicians unfamiliar with the distinctions (Letheby 1848–1849). At the scene, there may be transitory indications which if unnoticed there may be lost. An odour on the victim might suggest a poison, as with nicotine poisoning leaving a tobacco smell. A cherry red skin colour of the deceased might indicate carbon monoxide poisoning. Death certification procedures aim to provide safeguards, but much depends on the rigor of the procedures and on participants not 'cutting corners'.

M. Farrell, *Criminology of Homicidal Poisoning*,
DOI 10.1007/978-3-319-59117-9_9

Concealing Causes of Illness and Death

When a victim is ill, the perpetrator can deflect help or the possibility of someone ascertaining the symptoms by preventing relatives (or friends) from visiting. A poisoner can allay relative's concerns by suggesting that the illness is trivial, by inventing reasons why they should not visit, or if relatives are seldom in contact with the victim, simply not letting them know about the illness or even about the death when it occurs.

When unknowingly a physician is attending a patient who is being poisoned, the perpetrator can suggest an innocent cause of symptoms. Ethel Major [49] poisoned her unfaithful husband with strychnine, convincing the doctor that her spouse had epilepsy which he had kept secret to protect his job as a lorry/truck driver. The death certificate was duly completed showing cause of death as 'status epilepticus'. It was only when an anonymous letter alerted the authorities that the truth began to emerge.

Once a victim dies, the perpetrator may try to avoid an autopsy. This might be by disguising symptoms as natural causes, by suggesting that it was the deceased's wish, or if they are next of kin requesting themselves that there is no post-mortem examination. Where an autopsy takes place or where it is otherwise established that the deceased died of poisoning, the perpetrator may propose an innocent explanation. Perhaps the victim had an occupation or a hobby involving poison use. Environmental causes might be suggested where it is possible that poison such as lead could be ingested from the victim's immediate surroundings.

The crime scene may be arranged by the perpetrator and they might make subtle comments to suggest that suicide by poisoning was the cause of death. Kristin Rossum [82] used fentanyl to kill her husband Greg de Villers, elaborately arranging the scene to appear like suicide. If the victim had a drug abuse problem, it may be conveyed that a self-administered drug overdose caused death, rather than the perpetrator. It might be suggested that the victim accidentally or by suicide took an overdose of a drug that had been legitimately prescribed for them. For example, Florence Maybrick [21] poisoned her husband with the arsenic that he was taking medicinally. Reginald Hinks [48] gassed his father in law with carbon monoxide using an oven and claimed it was suicide. The perpetrator may maintain that the poison was administered by a third person, deliberately or accidentally. Relatedly, the poisoner can implicate another person as when Dorothea Waddingham [50] killed her nursing home patients with overdoses of morphine and claimed untruthfully that the visiting physician had provided the Home with surplus morphine tablets. Poison can be administered and the scene made to look like accidental death from another cause as when Kenneth Barlow [63] rendered his wife unconscious with insulin and drowned her in a bath to suggest accidental death. Similarly, Eugène Chantrelle [16] poisoned his wife with opium and stated that she died accidentally owing to a damaged gas main.

Death certification procedures may be evaded or abused. A physician may sign a death certificate of someone whom they (or an accomplice) have killed. The murdering physician may exploit the lack of experience of other doctors in endorsing death certification. Serial poisoner Dr. Edward Pritchard [12] killed his wife with antimony and aconite and certified death as gastric fever, later murdering his mother in law and certifying death as apoplexy. When Augusta Fullam [39] and Dr. Henry Clark killed Augusta's husband Edward, using arsenic to mimic the symptoms of heat stroke, Mrs Fullam administered the poison and Dr. Clark signed the death certificate.

Dr. Harold Shipman [81] killed, then used his medical knowledge to convince relatives that death was owing to various conditions rather than to anything suspicious. He also pressed for cremation so that evidence of the poison would not be available through exhumation. Having a single doctor practice further reduced any oversight or joint accountability. Furthermore, the detection process was not sufficiently rigorous when investigators examined concerns from a local physician of excessive deaths at Shipman's practice.

The perpetrator may press for a quick cremation making it more difficult to prove evidence of poisoning should suspicions arise later, although in the Graham Young [68] case evidence was presented of thallium being in cremated remains.

Physical Evidence of Poison and Its Destruction or Contamination

Detection of Physical Evidence

Physical evidence is collected from many sources. Crime scene samples may include clothing, finger and palm prints, bottles of medicine, hair and body tissue. Also evidence will come from: autopsy, exhumation, bodily specimens for analysis and forensic testing.

Sometimes, poison is found on the suspect on arrest. In 2010, Lakvir Singh [93] was convicted of secretly adding poison to a curry eaten by her former lover Lakhvinder Cheema. On her arrest, she was found in possession of the aconite that she had used. Graham Young [68] when arrested had thallium in his pockets with which he had been poisoning work colleagues. A bottle of Valentines' Meat Extract laced with arsenic was presented at the trial of Florence Maybrick [21] found guilty of poisoning her husband James and is displayed in the 'black museum' at Scotland Yard (Farrell 1998a). Physical traces of the poison may be detected on the deceased's clothing or nearby. Evidence of the poison being prepared or administered may be found on crockery, pans and other items.

Eliminating or Contaminating Physical Evidence

Most commonly, poison murder is perpetrated so that the death can appear accidental, suicidal, or owing to natural causes. Therefore, it is unusual for the body of a poison victim to be disposed of, a clear way of removing physical evidence. Never the less, in England, Roger and David Cooper [99] killed Sameena Imam with chloroform and buried her body in unoccupied ground. In fact, the perpetrators would have found it very difficult to make it appear that the death was natural, accidental, or suicidal and accordingly deposited the body, then conspired to create the illusion that Sameena had gone missing (West Midlands Police, private communication 2016).

A physician may attend a victim ill from poisoning while the perpetrator is apparently looking after them. If the doctor requests sample of vomit to be collected and kept, the perpetrator may not comply so that there is no physical evidence of the poison being administered. Attempts may be made to dispose of the poison used. Jeanne-Pierre Vaquier [45] killed his lover's husband with strychnine, and as the doctor attended the dying man, ran into the kitchen and removed a Bromo-salt bottle to which he had added the poison. He did not clean it thoroughly enough and traces of the poison were later detected. Charlotte Bryant apparently tried to burn the arsenical weed killer with which she had killed her husband but the charred tin container was recovered. An excessively tidy scene where there is a suspicious death may suggest that incriminating containers, dishes or cups have been cleaned or disposed of.

Exhumation and Autopsy and Their Subversion

Exhumation

Exhumation, the digging up of a previously buried body, is sometimes required in suspected poison cases to enable an autopsy. At the time of death and burial, crime may not have been suspected. Later, evidence may come to light or suspicions may form necessitating exhumation and autopsy. With repeat (and serial) poisoners, earlier poisonings may go undetected then suspicion may arise about a particular death and spread to earlier ones.

In the UK, and other jurisdictions informed by English law, the Coroner may order an exhumation of a body which is buried in their district should there be reason for the body to be examined. This may be to enable an inquest into the person's death, or in connection with any criminal proceedings relating to the death. Indeed the Coroner's role is important throughout homicide investigations and the Senior Investigating Officer and the Coroner (and their police and civilian officers) liaise closely (Association of Chief Police Officers/National Centre for Policing Excellence 2006 pp. 122–124).

In a typical exhumation, the grave and coffin are opened and identified. Where poisoning is suspected, samples of earth are taken from around the coffin as 'control' samples so that if poison such as arsenic is found in the body, it can be shown whether or not the substance had leached into the cadaver from grave earth.

Coffin and body are transferred for examination to a mortuary, where the pathologist, police, funeral director and forensic specialists may be present. Once the coffin is opened, samples of grave earth, coffin wood, coffin lining and shroud are taken to try to determine the possibility of contamination of the body after death with some toxic substance. If the body is badly decomposed, the pathologist has to exercise considerable skill to determine cause of death. Following exhumation, the body is reburied.

Avoiding Exhumation

A poisoner might avoid the consequences of a later exhumation by ensuring that the body is cremated. Where following a death, an individual presses urgently for cremation this might be for nefarious reasons. If a victim has been buried, should suspicions arise, exhumation may be requested by police or others. In retrospect, some poisoners could have avoided this had they not committed further crimes raising suspicion about earlier deaths.

In North Carolina in 1989 police investigating the illness of Reverend Dwight Moore, the second husband of Blanche Moore [78] found that he was suffering arsenic poisoning. Exhumation of the body of Blanche's boyfriend Raymond Reid revealed that he had died of arsenic poisoning years earlier, and Blanche was eventually sentenced to death for Reid's murder.

Autopsy

A forensic autopsy involves a Coroner as a judicial officer who investigates death in certain circumstances, usually referred by the police or a doctor. (In some US states the relevant person is a 'medical examiner'.) A death is referred if it

- occurred during or soon after a hospital procedure
- has an unknown cause
- is unexpected
- is violent, unnatural or suspicious, or
- is the result of an accident or an injury.

One purpose is to establish the mode or manner of death for example whether it was 'natural' or 'accidental', or the result of possible homicide. Another aim is to determine cause of death for example 'heart failure'. Time of death can be estimated although this is complicated by so many potential variables that pathologists tend to be cautious. Among features to consider are body temperature, ambient temperature of the surroundings and the extent of rigor mortice. Reviewing these findings, the pathologist decides whether to initiate an inquest (a legal investigation into the death) (Eliopulos 2003).

In criminal investigations, the deceased's body is examined as soon as possible to assist forensic investigation and to help determine cause of death. Where the death was a result of a violent confrontation or where a body was 'found' a preliminary examination is made at the scene including a visual examination of the corpse and its environment. Following this, the deceased is transported to the mortuary in a body bag.

Where death is from poisoning the scenario may differ. An individual may have been taken to hospital for treatment and may die there having been poisoned at home, so the 'crime scene' may not be secured. It may be some time before it is suspected that the location is a crime scene at all. John Armstrong [62] poisoned his baby Terence with Seconal sodium, and it was only following the autopsy that a police investigator interviewed the parents at home (where the baby had been murdered). Occasionally a case will involve a missing person inquiry and a 'found' body as with the remains found buried in the cellar of the house of Dr. Crippen [35] which was identified at the time as that of Cora Turner his wife.

Among people attending a forensic autopsy may be the pathologist, mortuary technician, detectives, scene of crime officers, fingerprint specialists, forensic scientists and police photographers. A video television team may record proceedings. Where possible, the body is identified by the family or relatives, although if a body is badly decomposed or disfigured, identification may be made through finger prints or familial DNA.

Clothing is examined and then removed and the external appearance of the body is noted. Certain signs taken in context may suggest poisoning. Alopecia (hair loss), white transverse lines across the nail bed and brittle nails may suggest chronic ingestion of heavy metal such as thallium, antimony, or arsenic. Pin point eye pupils may be caused by opiates like morphine. Conversely, dilated pupils can signal atropine, insulin or nicotine. Burns round the mouth suggest the ingestion of a corrosive such as acid.

Nail clippings and samples of hair may be taken. The body is then cleaned and incisions are made allowing scrutiny of internal organs. When the stomach is opened, signs of poisoning may be seen on the lining, such as adhering tablets, capsules or powder. Where poisoning is suspected, samples are taken for later analysis at the toxicology laboratory, for example from the stomach and its contents, liver, intestines, blood and urine. If morphine poisoning is possibility, the forensic laboratory will need samples of bile (a fluid, made in the liver and stored in the gallbladder, which breaks down fats to help their digestion). Skin and subcutaneous fat and muscle, and vitreous humour from the eye, are extracted where narcotic or insulin poisoning is suspected.

Following an initial autopsy cause of death may be determined as homicide and a suspect may be charged. Then defence lawyers, with the agreement of the

Coroner, arrange for another pathologist to conduct a 'defence autopsy' by arrangement with the first pathologist who may also attend.

Subverting Autopsy

As we have seen, autopsy is often instrumental in providing evidence of poisoning both in physical signs and in being part of a procedure yielding samples for forensic testing. Where autopsy can be subverted, then, an avenue of evidence can be closed. Given that the most decisive way is to avoid autopsy is to ensure that the body is cremated before it can be examined, indecent haste in an individual seeking to arrange this (physician, relative or others) may be nefarious.

A further way is to ensure that no suspicion arises that might necessitate an autopsy. This is possible where victims are elderly and death is expected. Where the perpetrator is a physician, their certifying cause of death can circumvent autopsy, as was the case with many of Dr. Harold Shipman's [81] patients. While certification of cause of death by an attending physician should always require the agreement of another doctor, procedures can become lax to the extent that this is a brief formality.

Forensic Testing and Its Evasion

Modern Toxicology

Pioneers heralding the modern era of toxicology include James Marsh (1789–1846) who devised a reliable test for the presence of minute amounts of arsenic (Farrell 1994a) and Jan Servais Stas (1813–1891) who discovered a test for vegetable poisons. Mathieu Orfila (1787–1853) is considered to be the founder of the modern discipline (Farrell 1994e). A range of techniques is available to contemporary toxicologists of which a few examples might be cited.

In chromatography ('thin layer', gas and high performance liquid) components of a mixture are physically separated by using the different distributions of each component between a 'stationary' phase and a 'mobile' phase. Radioimmunoassay measures the concentration of antigens (toxic bodies) such as blood hormone levels. It does this by using antibodies (blood proteins that attack antigens) that 'recognise' and attach themselves to specific sites on antigens, forming 'complexes'.

Atomic absorption spectroscopy detects whether elements (especially metallic ones) are present in a substance and may be used to trace mercury, lead, arsenic and similar, perhaps in a blood sample. In neutron activation analysis, a sample of material placed in a 'cyclotron' and bombarded with a huge neutron beam is changed into radioactive forms (isotopes) which will emit radiation enabling them to be identified by special instruments (see also Molina 2009, pp. 1–10).

Evading Forensic Testing for Poisons

Forensic tests are conducted not only on body fluids, waste products, tissues and other biological material (Gunn 2009) but also on other evidence which be incriminating. Any tampering with such material can impair a convincing evidence trail to the perpetrator and should raise suspicion.

Forensic testing is guided by the circumstances of a crime, their being neither time nor funding to undertake forensic 'fishing expeditions' for numerous suspected substances. Therefore, testing is guided by suspicions raised by police, pathologists, witnesses and others so that tests are conducted for specific substances. Perpetrators who are aware of this can use such knowledge. In the US, toxicologist Kristin Rossum [82] poisoned her husband Greg de Villers with fentanyl knowing that this substance was not routinely tested for at her laboratory. However, suspicions were raised around her husband's death and the investigations were contracted out to another laboratory where the relevant tests were made, contributing to Kristin's conviction.

Results of forensic testing can be evaded purely by a procedural mistake or, from the perpetrators viewpoint, by good luck. When Michael Barber died, it was thought to be owing to pneumonia and kidney failure, but pathologist David Evans was unconvinced. A request was made that samples of blood be sent to the National Poisons Unit in London and tested for the presence of Paraquat. When doctors later requested the results, they were informed that tests had eliminated this particular poison. This could have allayed any suspicions. However, Evans persisted. Further blood samples had been kept and these were sent to ICI the company which manufactured Paraquat and to the same National Poisons Unit in London. This time both sources came back with positive findings. It then became clear that the earlier sample had not been sent to the National Poisons Unit, and that the report of negative findings had been incorrect. It was to emerge that Susan Barber [71], Michael's wife, had put Paraquat in her husband's steak and kidney pie following an altercation about Susan's lover Richard Collins.

Motives: Revealing Them and Hiding Them

Revealing the Motives for Poison Murder

It is not always easy to determine a motive for crime, and several may interact. Motives for poison homicide cover the same spectrum as those for other murders (Farrell 1990a). Never the less, certain clusters are of interest: monetary gain/greed, escaping a relationship, jealousy and sadistic pleasure. A motive like driver can be 'factitious disorder imposed on another' (American Psychiatric Association 2013, pp. 324–327). A further factor may be that the perpetrator lacks the physical or emotional characteristics to murder in any other way although this is perhaps more of a constraint than a motive.

Greed/monetary gain as a motive was predominant in an analysis of 1026 mainly US and UK cases in which the offender was convicted of homicidal poisoning (Trestrail 2007) using an accepted crime classification (Douglas et al. 1992). Where motive was determined (about half of the cases) the commonest (21% of the whole 1026) was individual profit. With non-poisoning homicides, the perpetrator may kill the previously unknown victim in the course of a robbery. But with poison murder the victim is likely to be known to the killer and the gain may be from inheriting or life insurance. Greed motivated several spouse murders. Martha Marek [53] poisoned her husband and others for financial gain. Paul Marshall Curry [95], a US nuclear power plant engineer, killed his wife Linda with nicotine to claim life insurance money. In a strange variation of greed, Arthur Devereux [31] killed his wife and a son, partly to better financially provide for his remaining and favourite son. Greed was a motive in poisonings other than spouse murders. He Tiandai [101] a carer poisoned her victim He Yanzhu, a 70-year-old woman, in Guandong Province China using sleeping pills and dichlorvos. The reason was that the victim's family had agreed that if victim died before He Tiandai's monthly cheque was due, she would still be paid for the whole month. In India, an instance of poisoning for robbery (although not from complete strangers) involved K.D. Kempanna [94] killing six women temple worshipers with cyanide between 1997 and 2007, robbing them of money and valuables.

A seemingly common motive for poisoning is to *escape from a relationship*, including a marital one, perhaps to shake off tyranny; or to gain sexual freedom. Both may have been relevant when Major Herbert Armstrong [43] killed his overbearing wife and soon after took a philandering holiday. Charlotte Bryant [51], Edith Carew [26] and Maria Groesbeek [67] all poisoned their respective husbands to be with lovers. Marcus Marymont [65] killed his spouse with a view to seeing more of his mistress. Carlysle Harris [24] tired of his young clandestine wife and poisoned her. Killing to escape a spousal relationship seems to have declined in countries where legislation and public attitudes have made divorce and separation easier (Mason 1983).

Jealousy (sometimes expressed as revenge) has motivated poisonings. Cordelia Botkin [28] became the lover of a married man who later left his spouse. Trying to ensure that the wife did not pose a further threat, Cordelia mailed her rival poisonous chocolates. Jealousy led Infantry officer Adolph Hofrichter [36] to poison colleagues promoted above him. Linked with a desire for sexual exclusivity, jealousy appears to have motivated Lakvir Singh [93] to poison her lover Lakhvinder Cheema so that he could not marry his young fiancé. Under the perceived threat of his lover ending the relationship, Wei Entan [87] killed the woman's child with rat poison. Steven Roy Harper [69] used *N*-Nitrosodimethylamine to kill Duane Johnson and 11-month-old Chad (the husband and baby of Sandra Johnson, Harper's former girlfriend) from jealousy.

Sadistic pleasure can be linked to some poison murders partly by the nature of the deaths which can be particularly unpleasant and prolonged. George Chapman

[29] appears to have been motivated by sadism in committing a series of poison murders. Graham Young [68] killed several work colleagues, taking an intense interest in their sickness and symptoms which he had brought about. Norwegian nursing home manager Arnfinn Nesset [72] harboured sadistic motives in killing many of his patients. Martha Rendell [34] in Perth, Australia, swabbed the mouth of her stepson Arthur Morris with hydrochloric acid as a 'treatment' and was also suspected of killing her stepdaughters in a similar way. It was reported that she took great pleasure seeing the children in pain.

Regarding *factitious disorder imposed on another* (American Psychiatric Association 2013, pp. 324–327) this was previously known as 'factitious disorder by proxy'. In the UK, an alternative term 'fabricated or induced illness' may be used and sometimes the older term, 'Munchausen's syndrome by proxy'. Factitious here is used in the sense that the disorder is created and artificial rather than being real or 'natural'. This form of abuse, usually of a child, involves a parent or carer (typically the child's biological mother) causing or inventing symptoms of illness in the child in order to attract admiration or sympathy for themselves. The perpetrator may harm the victim to sustain the supposed illness (in line with our earlier discussion on theory about shaping of behaviour through rewards and sanctions). In a sense factitious disorder imposed on another has a built in reward for the perpetrator of the esteem and attention accruing to them. Genene Jones [74], a paediatric nurse, endangered the lives of the children in her care then sought adulation by 'saving' them, eventually killing children with injections of succinylcholine and other drugs. Lacey Spears [96] presented herself as a devoted mother whose son Garnett-Paul was frequently ill. In fact she was poisoning the child with salt, finally administering a lethal dose.

A *perpetrator may lack the physical or emotional characteristics to murder other than by poison.* This may help explain the choice of poison as a weapon but other motivations for murder would likely need to be proposed. Such a constraint may have applied to poisoners who killed and then fled the scene as with Quaker John Tawell [5] who poisoned his mistress with prussic acid, Dr. George Lamson [17] who killed his brother-in-law with aconite, and insurance seller Edward Black [44] who poisoned his wife Annie with arsenic. Perpetrators who mail poison to their victims may be unable to face carrying out the crime in any other way, as when farmer Walter Horsford [27] mailed strychnine to Annie Holmes who was pregnant with his child.

Hiding Motive

A motive of monetary gain/greed may be concealed by the perpetrator conveying that money is unimportant to them or that they have enough. It may take a careful examination of their financial affairs to indicate whether this is correct. In China, carer, He Tiandai [101] convinced her victim's family that she had simple country tastes and that money was not a priority until they noticed valuables missing and called the police who found the items concealed in the perpetrator's clothing.

Jealousy can be hidden if the perpetrator is discrete. The desire to escape from a relationship may be concealed by the perpetrator being solicitous towards the victim during their supposed illness and ensuring that witnesses see this. Sadistic pleasure may be also concealed by apparent solicitousness which is in fact the desire of the poisoner to see close up the victim's suffering.

Individuals with 'factitious disorder imposed on another' can be highly adept at hiding their motive under the pretence of being caring. Suspicions might be aroused where a parent or carer (including medical professionals) excessively appears at the centre of 'rescue' attempts or present themselves as suffering heroes. Where the victim was left alone at death or where poison was sent by mail this may indicate that a perpetrator lacks the physical or emotional characteristics to murder in any other way than by poison.

Poisoners have tried to conceal motive and murder by implicating a product and a manufacturer. A perpetrator kills a victim putting the poison in a well-known product, at the same time contaminating the same product in local shops, killing other people who consume it. The intention is that the initial murder will be mistakenly thought to be caused by the product being accidentally poisoned in its manufacture or distribution, or by someone else deliberately tampering with the product. In 1986, Stella Nickell [75] poisoned her husband Bruce with cyanide for life insurance. His death was thought to be owing to emphysema, a natural cause. As accidental death paid more than death from natural causes, it appears that Stella reported that her husband had died after having taken Excedrin capsules. To cover her story, she interfered with similar capsules in local stores. As a result, Susan Snow, a local bank manager died after taking the doctored capsules. Ultimately charged with product tampering Stella Nickel was sentenced to imprisonment (Trestrail 2007, pp. 22–23).

Knowledge, Access and Opportunity and Their Concealment

Knowledge of Poison and Where Obtained

A poisoner is expected to have some knowledge of poisons and their action perhaps gained through a profession or a hobby. Medics, pharmacist, farmers, pest controllers, horticulturalists, veterinarians and others will have knowledge of poisons and access to them. A particular hobby or interest such as chemistry will lead to knowledge of poisons.

Checking an individual's activities prior to a suspected murder by poisoning, police or others may find that the suspect has researched poisons in a local library or through the internet. The suspect may have spoken about their interest in poisons to others who may come forward as witnesses. Sometimes, perpetrators have given themselves away by taking an interest in poisons in their workplace as did Arthur Ford [60] the chemical firm administration manager with regard to cantharides.

Hiding Knowledge

Where the murder is extensively planned, computer searches for poisons and related matters may be wiped clean by the perpetrator or professionally. Books may be stolen from libraries or stores to avoid records being kept and later the books may be destroyed. Knowledge may be surreptitiously obtained through discussions with an innocent person or a clandestine collaborator.

Sometimes perpetrators have been caught by their making suspicious enquiries locally about the effects of poisons at a chemist, animal shelter or similar. However, where the perpetrator plans carefully they are able to make such enquiries less obviously and outside their local area where they are unlikely to be known.

Restrictions on Access to Poisons

Legislation has helped to restrict access to poisons including their sale and purchase. In Britain the *Arsenic Act 1851* controlled the sale of the poisons to the public. For example, it determined that anyone selling arsenic must record the sale in a book, following a set format. Subsequent Acts further restricted access to poisons (Farrell 1989c). In the US, pharmacies are legally required to keep and maintain a 'poison register' recording the poison sold, the amount, the stated use, date of purchase, and the buyer's name and address (Trestrail 2007, p. 44).

Certain trends are discernible. Poisons have been identified (for example by specifying them in an agreed list). Gradually the sale and distribution of those poisons have been restricted to people with particular qualifications, or with legitimate reasons for their use. Concurrently, clearer roles and responsibilities have developed for physicians, pharmacists and other medically related professions in relation to access to and distribution of poisons. Records have been required of the sale and purchase of such poisons.

Detection is aided where records are kept confirming that a suspect has purchased poison. When Frenchman Jean-Pierre Vaquier [45] killed his lover's husband with strychnine, investigators established that he had bought the substance at a chemist in London, signing for it under the name 'Wanker'. In Cornwall, England, Edward Black [44] having poisoned his wife with arsenic was found to have signed a poison register at a St. Austell chemist.

Evading Restrictions on Access to Poisons

Poisons can be made from plants so long as the instruments for preparing the poison are concealed. Count Hippolyte de Bocarme [6] killed his brother-in-law with nicotine but left in his cellar the requisite distilling equipment. An easily available poison for example antifreeze can be stolen from a store or a neighbour's garage, leaving no record of purchase. Access to poisons may be through a person's occupation as with medical personnel and related professions possessing drugs.

As Trestrail (2007) points out poisons can also be obtained from laboratories whether medical, educational (schools and colleges) or industrial. Hobbies such as traditional (non-digital) photography, minerology and jewellery making can also involve the use of poisonous substances. Antique drug and chemical bottles may be sold with their contents still in place on the misguided assumption that because the contents are old, they are harmless (Ibid. pp. 42–44). As well poisons being available from such sources, they may also be stolen.

Opportunity to Administer Poison

Often when poison is administered the poisoner is physically present, giving the victim the substance in food or drink. For example, Ryan Furlough [86] gave cyanide to his friend Benjamin Vassilev in a soft drink. In Indonesia, Jessica Wongso [100] was in a café with Wayan Salihin when she poisoned her with cyanide. In other instances, the poison may be given under the guise of a medical procedure, perhaps as a drug overdose as with many medical poisonings.

Concealing Opportunity to Administer Poison

Trying to take advantage of the expectation that the poisoner is physically present when poison is administered, several poisoners have mailed poison to their intended victim. Farmer Walter Horsford [27] killed Mrs. Holmes (pregnant with his child) with strychnine mailed to her with instructions to take it. There is the risk that the wrong person or other people in addition to the victim will consume the poison. Cordelia Botkin [28] mailed arsenic impregnated chocolates to her lover's wife, Mary Dunning, killing her victim, but also inadvertently poisoning Mary's sister who shared the confections.

A strange attempt at concealment involved Dr. George Lamson [17] who killed his young brother-in-law Percy John with aconite in a Dundee cake while visiting him at his school in Wimbledon, England. The pair was joined by the school principal, and Lamson passed round ready cut pieces of his cake ensuring that Percy took the single poisoned piece. The killer made a great pantomime of producing some capsules and filling one of them with sugar which he gave to Percy as a medicine. Ten minutes after Lamson departed, Percy fell ill, dying the same night. Presumably, the rigmarole with the cake and the 'medicine' was to move any suspicion to the capsules, which were innocent, a case of attempted concealment in plain sight. Another aspect of the plan was that the murderer would be absent when death occurred.

Conclusion

A poisoner can mask a victim's cause of death. When a victim is ill, help or the ability of someone finding out about the symptoms can be deflected by the perpetrator deterring or preventing relatives or friends from visiting. A perpetrator can suggest to the attending physician a spurious yet credible cause of symptoms of poisoning. When victim dies, the poisoner may try to avoid autopsy by disguising symptoms as natural causes, by suggesting that it was the deceased's wish, or if they are next of kin protesting autopsy themselves. Where it is established that the deceased died of poisoning, the perpetrator may propose that suicide by poisoning was the cause of death, and arrange the crime scene accordingly. If the victim had a drug problem, a self-administered drug overdose can be mooted as cause of death. The perpetrator may claim that the poison was administered by a third person, deliberately or accidentally. A physician signing a death certificate of someone whom he has killed, or in collusion with an accomplice who has killed, can disguise nefarious practices. The murdering physician may also use an inexperienced doctor to confirm cause of death, or convince relatives that death was natural. Lack of rigour in the detection process can thwart an arrest.

A wide range of physical evidence can aid proof of poisoning. The poison itself, or traces of it are clearly potentially incriminating. An excessively tidy scene may suggest that otherwise suspect containers have been cleaned or discarded.

A poisoner might attempt avoid the consequences of a later exhumation by pressing for cremation of the victim, although there is still the possibility of later identifying poison traces in the ashes. Following a poisoning where no suspicion arose the later poisoning of a further victim using the same modus operandi has sometimes revealed the earlier offence.

Autopsy often provides evidence of poisoning both through physical signs and through being part of the procedure by which samples are sent for forensic testing. Where autopsy can be subverted an avenue of evidence can be closed. The perpetrator can avoid suspicion by setting the scene for an apparently expected death because the victim is elderly or because 'illness' has been created by chronic poisoning. Corrupted death certification procedures when a physician is the perpetrator can evade autopsy. Autopsy at a later date is denied if the perpetrator ensures that the deceased is cremated.

Forensic procedures can be subverted by the poisoner tampering with or destroying potential evidence such bodily fluids passed when the victim was alive.

Any mistake in the forensic procedures or poor communication between departments can enable the murderer to evade suspicion.

Among motives for poisoning are monetary gain/greed, escaping a relationship, jealousy and sadistic pleasure. A motive-like driver is factitious disorder imposed on another. Additional to such motives a constraining factor may be that the perpetrator lacks the physical or emotional characteristics to murder in any other way. Extreme measures can be taken to hide motive such as product tampering to conceal a poisoning.

Some poisoners by the nature of their work are already highly knowledgeable of poisons. Where a murder has to gain knowledge of a poison, there may be evidence such as witness to whom they spoke, computer files, records of library loans, purchases of book and so on. However, the poisoner might avoid speaking to others of poison, might have computer records professionally wiped and might steal or otherwise clandestinely acquire books or other sources.

Poisoners need to plan to gain access to noxious substances without leaving a trail. An easily available poison can be stolen, so leaving no record of purchase. Poisons can be made from naturally occurring plants if preparations are concealed. They may be acquired through a person's occupation as with the access of medical and related personnel to drugs. Poisons can also be obtained from different kinds of laboratories. Hobbies can also involve the use of toxic substances. Antique drug and chemical bottles may be misguidedly sold with their contents in place. Poisons can also be stolen.

Opportunity to administer the poison can be disguised. For example, poison can be mailed to a victim, although this risks the wrong person or other people in addition to the victim consuming it. The poisoner may attempt to conceal the poison in plain sight.

Suggested Activity

Work through the sections of the ACPO/CENTREX (2006) *Murder Investigation Manual* or your closest national equivalent. Note implications for strategic management, operations and tactics where a poison homicide might have occurred.

Further Reading

Association of Chief Police Officers/National Centre for Policing Excellence. (2006). *Murder investigation manual 2006* ACPO/CENTREX.

The manual systematically covers the strategic management of investigations; and operations and tactics for homicide investigation.

Trestrail, J. H. (2007). *Criminal poisoning: investigational guide for law enforcement, toxicologists, forensic scientists and attorneys* (2nd ed.). Totowa, NJ: Humana Press

A broad ranging book, engagingly written.

References

American Psychiatric Association. (2013). *Diagnostic and statistical manual of mental disorders fifth edition (DSM5).* Washington DC: APA.

Association of Chief Police Officers/National Centre for Policing Excellence. (2006). *Murder investigation manual 2006.* ACPO/CENTREX.

Douglas, J. E., Burgess, A. W., Burgess, A. G. (1992). *Crime classification manual.* New York: Lexington Books.

Eliopulos, L. N. (2003). *The Death Investigator's Handbook: Volume 3—Scientific Investigations.* Boulder, Colorado: Paladin Press.

Farrell, M. (1989c). 'Arsenic Poisoning: The Role of Legal Controls'. *Solicitors Journal, 133*(35), 1101–1102.

Farrell, M. (1990). What's your Poison? *Solicitors Journal, 134*(29), 825.

Farrell, M. (1994a). 'Pioneer forensic toxicologists: marsh orfila and their predecessors'. *The Criminologist, 18*(1), 33–36.

Farrell, M. (1994b). 'Pioneer forensic toxicologists: taylor stas, tardieu and selmi'. *The Criminologist, 18*(3), 141–145.

Farrell. (1998a). 'Poisoner of the Black Museum'. *The Criminologist, 22*(1), 35–41.

Gunn, A. (2009) *Essential forensic biology* (2nd ed.). Chichester, UK and New Jersey, US: Wiley-Blackwell.

Letheby, H. (1848–1849) 'On the probability of confounding cases of arsenical poisoning with those of cholera'. *Pharmaceutical Journal, 8*, 237–240.

Mason, J. K. (1983) *Forensic medicine for lawyers* (2nd ed.) London: Butterworths.

Molina, D. K. (2009). *Handbook of forensic toxicology for medical examiners* (Practical Aspects of Criminal and Forensic Investigations Series) New York: Taylor and Francis/CRC Press.

Trestrail, J. H. (2007) *Criminal poisoning: investigational guide for law enforcement, toxicologists, forensic scientists and attorneys* (2nd ed.). Totowa, NJ: Humana Press.

West Midlands Police. (2016). Private communication.

Westveer, A. E., Trestrail, J. H., & Pinizotto, J. (1996). Homicidal poisonings in the United States —an analysis of the uniform crime reports from 1980 through 1989. *American Journal of Forensic Medicine and Pathology, 17*(4), 282–288.

Chapter 10
Poisoners on Trial

Introduction

Overviews of criminal court procedures are provided by Sprack (2011) in relation to England and Wales and, regarding the US, by Hemmens et al. (2017). Here we focus on issues arising in trials concerning poison homicide. In England, the crime of poisoning was specifically included in law under the *Offences Against the Person Act 1861*. Section 23 of the Act dealt with endangering life or causing grievous bodily harm by poisoning. Even the intention to annoy was included (Section 24). While no distinction was made between a drug and a poison, in the case of drugs, the dose and its mode of presentation were central to the definition. For example, the issue of whether or not the drug takes the form of a reputable pharmaceutical preparation may be crucial. Also, the intention of the user is important (In Scotland, the situation is different, poisoning being a crime under common law).

For proof of murder by poison, it needs to be shown that.

- the deceased died from poisoning
- the accused administered the fatal dose
- the accused intended to kill (or grievously harm) the victim in doing so.

Towards the Trial

The common law systems of the US, Canada, Australia, and England and Wales, and the hybrid system of Scotland are underpinned by the 'adversary' principle. In civil law systems such as in France, the underpinning is 'inquisitorial'. A basic characteristic of the adversary principle is that it involves a search for proof, but lacks transparency because each side guards its own evidence. On the other hand the inquisitorial principle involves a search for truth but lacks impartiality because of the great trust placed in the investigator (Sanders and Young 2012, pp. 838–839).

M. Farrell, *Criminology of Homicidal Poisoning*,
DOI 10.1007/978-3-319-59117-9_10

In fact, the situation is more subtle than this characteristic suggests. For example, there are rules of disclosure that prevent the suppression of certain relevant evidence.

Another distinction is between, a model of 'due process' and one of 'crime control'. Values associated with *due process* prioritise civil liberties in order to increase the chances of the innocent being acquitted but at the risk of acquitting many guilty people. They rigorously control the actions and effects of crime control agencies. *Crime control* values, on the other hand, put the conviction of the guilty first, but risks convicting some innocents and infringing the civil liberties of some citizens. They do not as rigorously control the actions and effects of crime control agencies (Sanders and Young 2012, pp. 838–839).

An adversarial relationship is initiated when police challenge a suspected person. Due process protections come into play such as cautioning against incriminating one's self. On arrest when a suspect may be taken to a police station and detained, may be interrogated and have their home searched, due process protections include the right of access to a lawyer. At prosecution, the accused has the protection of legal representation. Securing a conviction requires yet more evidence. For conviction, the proof is not required to be absolute, but 'beyond reasonable doubt' (Sanders and Young 2012, p. 839). Where there is insufficient proof, the accused is acquitted irrespective of whether guilty in actuality. In effect as the suspect, later the accused, moves closer to trial, protections of due process are increased. The burden of proof lies with the prosecution who must make the jury sure of guilt.

A distinction may be made between 'direct evidence' which involves eyewitness accounts and which may or may not be reliable (Loftus 1996), and 'circumstantial evidence' which requires inference to make it applicable. In some instances, a long time may elapse between police challenging a suspect and that person being arrested. In part, this is because of the nature of poison cases which can involve much circumstantial evidence and witnesses who at the time did not realise that they were witnessing a crime. US police had suspicions about Lynn Turner [88] who killed her former husband with antifreeze in, but it was years later when she similarly poisoned her boyfriend that these crystallised sufficiently for them to be able to make an arrest and secure conviction.

If the due process is followed and the prosecutors are confident that there is sufficient evidence to give the chance of conviction, the case moves to court. Issues that may then arise are the subject of the remainder of this chapter.

Establishing that the Deceased Died from Poisoning

Was Death Owing to Natural Causes?

Often, indications of poison have been mistaken for symptoms of illness. When Major Armstrong killed his wife with arsenic, it was thought that she had died of a wasting condition. Comte de Bocarme [6] claimed that his brother in law had suffered a fatal seizure when in reality the aristocrat had given him a lethal dose of nicotine. At the trial of Florence Maybrick [21] for the murder of her husband James with arsenic it was claimed (unsuccessfully) that his death was from natural causes and that the poisons found in his body were the self-administered doses of a hypochondriac.

Confounding poison murder with death from an illness was a feature of several cases in which physicians were perpetrators. Dr. Carl Coppolino [66] poisoned Colonel Farber (the husband of his mistress) with succinylcholine chloride and death was certified as coronary thrombosis. When Dr. Phillip Cross's [20] wife was dying from the arsenic that he was administering her, he diagnosed her as suffering from typhoid, being careful to get a second opinion from a young, newly qualified doctor who concurred. In a similar fashion Dr. Henry Clark [39] arranged the poisoning of his lover's husband with arsenic, he certified death as being due to heat stroke.

Where There Indications of Poisoning When the Deceased Was Dying?

The victim themselves may express concerns and suspicions if there is anyone to listen to them. Before he died, Lakhvinder Cheema (correctly) told relatives that his former lover Lakvir Singh [93] had poisoned him. Where there were witnesses as the victim was dying, they may report symptoms that suggest poisoning. During the trial of Catherine Wilson [10] for the murder of Maria Soames with colchicum seeds, Dr. Taylor called by the prosecution stated that the deceased's symptoms were consistent with those of colchicum poisoning. Another doctor was called. He had attended James Dixon a former lover of Catherine when Dixon had died, it appeared from natural causes. This second doctor stated that with hindsight the symptoms were consistent with colchicum poisoning.

Is There Physical Evidence of the Suspected Poison Being Administered to the Deceased?

If it is claimed that a certain poison has been used, it is helpful if physical indications can be shown such as traces of arsenic in the deceased's hair and nails. There may be a debate about whether or not any poison found in the corpse after exhumation got there by other means than the deceased being poisoned in life. It may be claimed that the poison has been introduced for example from grave earth, the coffin constituents, or artefacts interred with the body.

At the trail of Dr. Robert Buchanan [25], who killed his wife at their New York home, an example arose of the importance of such physical evidence. Prosecution lawyers claimed that Buchanan had killed his wife with morphine, a decisive indicator of which is that the eyes contract to pinpoints. Yet as the defence pointed out, although autopsy indicated the presence of morphine, the important tiny eye pupils were not evident. In turn, the prosecution team called witnesses to attest that Buchanan had boasted that he could counteract the effect of morphine on the eyes by introducing drops of belladonna. It a dramatic demonstration to the court, a cat was killed with morphine, its eyes treated with drops of belladonna, and the eye pupils found after the animal's death to be dilated.

Can It Be Established that the Accused Administered the Fatal Dose?

The Accused Was not Present When Death Occurred

It may appear a reasonable line of defence to show that the alleged poisoner was not present when the victim died, but this is not necessarily convincing. Normally it would be expected that a murderer is present at the death of the victim but not always. When a murderer plants an explosive device with a time delay he is unlikely to be in the vicinity when the death takes place. Poisoners too have ensured that they are not present when death takes place for example by mailing poison to the victim.

Farmer Walter Horsford [27] killed his cousin a widow Mrs. Holmes with strychnine sent to her through the post with instructions to take it. At his trial, a handwriting specialist was called. He testified that a letter and writing on two packages containing strychnine that had been found in Mrs. Holmes's house were both written by Horsford. Both packages had been found under the deceased's feather bed. On one package had been written, 'One dose, take as told'. On the other package which contained a few crystals having been apparently taken was written, 'Take in a little water. 'Tis quite harmless. Will come in a day or two'. The letter found in the downstairs section of the house said that the writer would come on Friday to make arrangements, that he did not wish to write again, and did not wish his wife to know.

Adolph Hofrichter [36], Marie Lafarge [4], and Cordelia Botkin [28] are further examples of absent poisoners. In such instances the same proofs can apply as with cases when the perpetrator is present. It can still be shown that the victim died of poisoning, that it was effectively administered (at a distance) by the perpetrator, and that the perpetrator intended to kill.

The Accused Was not in Possession of the Implicated Poison

If is to be demonstrated that the accused administered the fatal dose of poison, but there is no evidence that the accused had ever possessed poison, the prosecution case becomes more difficult. Therefore it is helpful to be able to show that the accused did possess poison.

In the killing of baby Terence Armstrong with Seconal sodium, his parents were suspected but denied ever having had the drug in their home. It emerged however that five months before Terence had died, at the Royal Navy hospital where John Armstrong [62] the baby's father worked, a dangerous drugs cupboard had been rifled. Among the stolen items was Seconal sodium in capsules.

The Accused Was in Possession of Poison but Had a Legitimate Reason

If it is evident that the accused was or had been in possession of the poison, a defence can be that there was a reason for its possession other that any intention to harm the victim. Providing reasons for being in possession of poison, sometimes relates to their legitimate use. Medical personnel have the readiest explanation for possessing certain poisons as they may be used medicinally in small doses and be kept as part of their medical supplies. Dr. Harold Shipman [81] and Dr. Robert Buchanan [25] had access to the morphine that they used for murder. As a medical student, Carlysle Harris [24] who got rid of his wife with the drug had ready access to morphine. Manager of a nursing home, Dorothea Waddingham [50] used morphine to kill patients, claiming that she had administered it on doctor's instructions. Dentist Dr. Etiene Deschamps [23] killed his child victim with the chloroform that he legitimately used in his practice.

It may be unnecessary to provide a plausible reason for possessing poison when it is part of everyday life. This was the case when Reginald Hinks [48] gassed his father-in-law in a domestic gas oven and tried to pass the death off as suicide. Florence Maybrick [21] killed her husband with arsenic which she claimed was intended for cosmetic use. After killing his lover's husband with strychnine, Jean Pierre Vaquier [45] stated that he had bought the substance to use in wireless experiments. Poisoner Johann Hoch [32] when found with a pen containing arsenic in his possession claimed that it was intended for his own suicide.

In fact, the very reason that an accused was made the subject of suspicion can also be reinterpreted as a defence. The accused may have legitimately possessed a poison in connection with a hobby or their work, but can argue that although they possessed it, they did not administer poison to the victim.

Was Death Accidental?

Evidence that is presented by the prosecution will include that the cause of death of the supposed victim was by poisoning. Alternative explanations are sometimes offered either in a statement made to police or others by the suspect, or in legal pleas at the trial. These relate to the nature of poisoning as opposed to other modus operandi. Where the weapon has been a gun, knife, or blunt instrument, then signs of violence that are usually apparent on the body make certain defences plausible, that the shooting was accidental or that the weapon was used in self-defence. In the case of poisoning, external signs are not always clearly evident, except perhaps where the substance was injected, leaving puncture marks, or where the poison was so corrosive that burn marks were left on the victim's mouth and nose. Absence of external marks of violence leave it open to the poisoner to suggest that death was from another cause, hoping that the real cause will not be established. Accordingly, after poisoning his wife with opium, Eugène Chantrelle [16] stated that a gas leak was responsible.

Claiming that death was due to a cause other than murder can be a reasonable defence even if the poison found in the body is available for medicinal and other uses. Florence Maybrick [21] claimed that the arsenic in her husband's body was the result of his taking it as a tonic.

Mary Wilson [64] was accused of murdering Oliver Leonard (her second husband) and Ernest Wilson (her third husband) with elemental phosphorus. Rose Heilbron (Later Mrs. Justice Heilbron) led the defence and questioned Dr. Ian Barclay the Director of the Home Office Forensic Science Laboratory, Gosforth. He stated that the only source that he knew of elemental phosphorus outside of laboratories was in rat poison and beetle poison. Miss Heilbron pointed out that yellow phosphorus pills were on the lists of five well-known manufacturing chemists. One example was damiana pills which were used as an aphrodisiac. The implication of this point was to suggest that Oliver Leonard and Ernest Wilson were taking damiana pills to improve their sexual performance. This leaves open the possibility that the deceased took too many pills by accident. However, the prosecution led by Geoffrey Veale argued that the amount of phosphorus found in the bodies suggested taking about 150 pills, which it was inconceivable to think could be done by accident. In the event Mary Wilson was found guilty (It was surmised that she had administered the poison in cough mixture to disguise the taste).

Was the Cause of Death Suicide?

Arguing that death was suicide has been a defence in several notable cases. Knocking his father-in-law to the floor and bruising the old man's head, Reginald Hinks [48] then put the victim's head in the gas oven to kill him. He claimed in his defence that the old man had committed suicide and that the bruises were sustained as Hinks had tried to revive him.

When Major Herbert Armstrong [43] was tried for the murder of his wife Katherine, the defence led by Sir Henry Curtis Bennett K.C. argued that Katherine had committed suicide with a single dose of arsenic. But there was a discrepancy between the single dose theory and the time that it should have taken for the poison to reach part of the body where it had been detected at autopsy. To try to meet this difficulty, the defence called Dr. Toogood to state that most of the arsenic had become encysted on the stomach wall. Reference was made to the case of the Duc de Praslin in which a similar claim was made. Mr. Justice Darling in his summing up, returned to the Duc de Praslin case, pointing out that it had involved falsified evidence.

In the trial of toxicologist Kristin Rossum [82], convicted of poisoning her husband Greg de Villiers with the opiate drug fentanyl for which she was sentenced in 2002, the defence argued that de Villiers was suicidal and had poisoned himself. Prosecution lawyers maintained that he had been killed by his wife for two reasons. The first was to prevent him revealing to her work managers at the San Diego County Medical Examiner's Office that she was having an affair with the head toxicologist Michael Robertson. The second reason was to stop him revealing that she was using metaphine stolen from the coroner's laboratory. Greg's brother Jerome de Villiers also testified that it was hard to believe that Greg had committed suicide in the alleged way because Greg hated taking drugs.

Can It Be Established that the Accused Both Administered the Poison and Intended to Kill the Victim?

Did the Accused Administer the Poison but not Intend to Kill?

Intent is effectively a subjective state of mind and so not easy to prove, but may be inferred from certain evidence. Prior to the death the accused may have threatened to kill the victim or expressed a desire to do them serious harm. Evidence may be uncovered of premeditation and detailed planning, a feature often considered part and parcel of poison murder. In non-poison homicides, the accused can have an argument with the victim, grab an item that happens to be close at hand, strike the victim with it and kill them and yet still claim that there was no intent to kill. But to put a lethal dose of poison, bought some time earlier into a victim's food or drink does not lend itself to an argument that it was done on the spur of the moment.

However, even when the accused has admitted administering the poison, there is room to claim that death was not intended. Dr. Etienne Deschamps [23] killed a 12-year-old girl whom he had periodically been sexually abusing. Having poisoned her with chloroform, his defence was that he had given the child an accidental overdose. Arthur Ford [60], office manager of a manufacturing chemist, gave sweets laced with cantharides which he thought was an aphrodisiac to a secretary with whom he was infatuated killing her (and another secretary who also took a doctored sweet). He was convicted of manslaughter rather than murder because the court considered that he had no intention to kill. Maria Groesbeek [67] claimed to have given her husband the ant poison which killed him only to make him so ill that he would grant her a divorce. In the US in 2003, Daniel Bondeson [83], a New

Sweden potato farmer killed Walter Morrill a 78-year-old fellow church worshiper with arsenic. Bondeson committed suicide five days later leaving a confessional note saying that he only intended to harm members of the church after an internal dispute.

A variation of the idea that the perpetrator did not intend to kill was seen at the trail of nursing home manager Dorothea Waddingham [50] tried for the poisoning by morphine of Ada Baguley a former resident of the home. Waddingham tried at Nottingham Assizes, testified that she had indeed given the morphine, but that it had been on the instructions of Dr. Mansfield who attended the resident. The doctor however when called as a witness, convincingly denied giving any such instructions.

Was the Accused Insane?

Demonstrating an intention to kill implies that the accused was responsible for his or her actions. If it can be shown that the accused is insane, this constitutes a defence. Partial insanity was the defence of Sadamichi Hirasawa [56] when he robbed a bank and killed the staff with cyanide pellets. He claimed that his insanity had been caused by an anti-rabies injection given to him years before the offence. This plea was not upheld and he was found guilty. Chemist's assistant Arthur Deveureux [31], who poisoned his wife and twin sons, tried to feign insanity at his trial but was unsuccessful in convincing the court and was found guilty.

Dr. Arthur Waite [40] was tried and entered a plea of not guilty but in evidence to the court admitted killing his mother and father-in-law for their money. At appeal he pleaded insanity, claiming to have a dual personality, half of which was an Egyptian acquaintance of Queen Cleopatra. Doctors were called to concur with a diagnosis of insanity but the jury, unimpressed, returned a verdict of guilty and Waite was subsequently executed.

However, the trial of Teresa Conroy [57] was a different matter. She killed her son with coal gas and an overdose of his epilepsy medication before placing the corpse in a mattress where it was soon after discovered by the boy's father. At her trial before Mr. Justice Havers at the Old Bailey, a verdict of guilty but insane was returned and Conroy was detained for an indefinite period.

Other Issues

The Character of the Perpetrator

Poisoners seem to be held in particular abhorrence by society at large, media responses to poisonings often reflecting this. Consequently, where someone is standing trial for alleged poisoning it is especially helpful if the accused can be presented in such a positive light that they could not be suspected of so terrible a crime. Conversely the prosecution is eager to reveal that the defendant has it in their character to perpetrate poisoning. A vivid example of this arose in the trail of Frederick Seddon [37], a district superintendent of an assurance company, who was accused (with his wife) of killing their lodger Eliza Barrow with arsenic. Sir Edward Marshall Hall K.C., defending argued that Miss Barrow had died of chronic arsenic poisoning (presumably self-administered) not through acute arsenic poisoning administered by Seddon as the prosecution alleged. He made a strong point when Sir William Wilcox the Home Office (government nominated) pathologist had to admit that traces of arsenic had been found in Eliza Barrow's hair. This suggested that arsenic may have been taken up to a year prior to death. (Overnight Wilcox conducted an experiment that suggested that the arsenic in the hair may have come from fluid found in Miss Barrow's coffin). But a key feature of Seddon's evidence was the negative impression that he conveyed (with the help of the prosecution led by the Attorney-General Sir Rufus Isaacs). Isaacs who specialised in commercial cases painstakingly worked through the transactions between Seddon and Eliza Barrow. Miss Barrow had held stocks, leasehold interests, cash and other assets which over a period of eight months, she had gradually signed over to Seddon for a fairly generous annuity. Frederick Seddon's, lack of fellow feeling and his obsession with money was glaringly clear as he worked through in his cross-examination the tiny details of the transactions. This along with a range of other evidence led the jury after retiring for only an hour to return a verdict of guilty on Frederick Seddon and not guilty on his wife.

More recently in England, 'bad character evidence' and the rules for admitting or precluding it are covered in the Criminal Justice Act 2003, section 101. In the US, the supposed character of an alleged murderer was a feature of the trail of Cynthia Sommer which initially found her guilty of poisoning her husband an offence of which she was later acquitted (Perry 2008). In San Diego, in 2002 the 23-year-old marine Todd Sommer became ill and died soon after with the cause of death certified as a heart attack. The following year, military authorities tested tissue preserved from Todd's autopsy and were said to have found lethal levels of arsenic. Authorities took the view that Cynthia Sommer had killed her husband to gain insurance and survivor benefits. She was arrested and stood trial in 2007 in California. Although the trial judge had ruled that the prosecution could not reveal the behaviour of the widow following Todd's death, defence counsel raised the matter when presenting Cynthia as a grieving widow. Rebutting this, the prosecution then presented evidence that in the weeks following Todd's death Cynthia had had breast implants, had sexual relations with different partners, thrown parties, and moved to Florida with a new boyfriend. Prosecutors also stated that Sommer had made enquiries about money only hours after her husband's death. Found guilty of first degree murder in January 2007, Sommer filed for a new trial and followed up an issue that had arisen during trial about the unreliability of laboratory results. A retrial was held in May 2008 with a new defence attorney who requested insistently that the prosecution produce the tissues that remained from Todd's autopsy. Prosecutors maintained that no such tissue existed but after the defence made a formal discovery demand, the tissues were found. When test was carried out on these samples including liver and kidney, they were found to be negative for arsenic. Based on these finding the prosecution requested that the court dismiss the charges, and Sommer was released.

The Role and Credibility of Witnesses

Where there is a violent altercation between two people in the course of which one kills the other say with a gun, knife or punches, any witnesses are clear that violence is taking place. They are likely to register strong impressions of what happened. Of course the accuracy of these can still be challenged. But poisoning is often a silent and secret killing of which the victim is unaware and which others may not even realise that they are witnessing.

Therefore the memory of witnesses may be less vivid that with other crimes. If the poisoning is chronic and the victim is ill over an extended period, suspicions may be aroused and the alertness of witness may be sharpened. But where this does not happen, witness may be put in the position of being asked to recall things that they have no cause to remember because the events were not seen as unusual or suspicious when first encountered.

Technical Evidence

In poison trials the emphasis is on explaining as clearly as possible the complex information demonstrating that the crime took place. While technical forensic evidence can be important in other homicide trials, in poisoning cases, by the nature of the modus operandi important technical evidence is likely to be presented to the court. This may concern the poison itself: the qualities such as what it looks like, its smell and taste, its action, the symptoms that it causes, and its distribution in and elimination from the body. Where a corpse has been exhumed, evidence will need to cover the possibility that poisonous substances may have entered the body from the grave environment rather than having been administered to the victim in life.

In the trial of nurse Charles Higgs [90] in 2006 the importance of a 'trace' of poison and the knowledge of the accused was raised in evidence about the poison and its administration. Higgs was ultimately convicted of killing his wife former State Controller Kathy Augustine with an injection of succinylcholine chloride. In arguments about the evidence of the drug in the victim's body, the defence lawyer David Houston sought to equate the idea of a trace with their being little evidence to convict. He stated, 'I'm not really sure what a trace is, but it's certainly not enough to convict somebody beyond a reasonable doubt of murder'. The defence also raised questions about the way that the drug had been administered. The site of injection was the muscle of the buttocks. But being a nurse, Higgs would have known that the drug acts intravenously and would not have been expected to use a muscle site for the injection. Prosecutor Tom Barb pointed out. 'Succinylcholine is not a recreational drug. If that is present, somebody put it in her. The only one to put it in her was her husband'.

A complicated picture of toxicological, medical and related evidence arose in the trial of Dr. Robert Ferrante [97]. In 2013, University of Pittsburgh neuroscientist Dr. Robert Ferrante, telephoned 911 as his wife neurologist Dr. Autumn Klein was ill. She was taken to University of Pittsburgh Medical Centre Presbyterian Hospital where doctors tried over three days to save her life. During that period blood samples were taken and as a preliminary analysis showed high acid levels the physician ordered toxicological tests for cyanide poisoning. The results did not come through until after Dr. Klein had died and her body had been cremated. No autopsy was held. When the test results were available they indicated lethal levels of cyanide.

In 2005, Dr. Ferrante stood trial for the murder of his wife. Prosecution was led by Assistant Allegheny County District Attorney Lisa Pelligrini alleged that Ferrante had killed his wife with cyanide. It emerged that Dr. Klein wanted another child and Ferrante did not. The prosecutor stated that Dr. Ferrante also thought that his wife was having an affair. It was stated that the poison was bought through his work ostensibly for experiments relating to his stem cell research into Lou Gehrig's disease. He added the cyanide to his wife's fertility boosting energy drink. It was revealed that Ferrante made online searches for cyanide poisoning and how it might be detected by autopsy after death. In prosecution medical evidence, Dr. Christopher Holstege of the University of Virginia testified that the victim's symptoms excluded everything but cyanide poisoning.

For the defence, attorney William Difenderfer called Dr. Robert Middleberg, vice president of a private crime laboratory in Pennsylvania who stated that tests on Dr. Klein's blood carried out at his laboratories were inconclusive. Similar testimony was given by Dr. Shaun Carstairs of the San Diego Naval Medical Centre and by Dr. Cyril Wecht a forensic pathologist. As well as this conflicting toxicological testimony, Difenedefer drew attention to the circumstantial nature of much of the evidence and the lack of an autopsy.

Strong points for the prosecution were the cross-examination of Dr. Ferrantes which revealed many inconsistencies in his statements to the authorities. Also the jury were played a recording of the emergency 911 call by Ferrante in which Autumn Klein could be heard in the background apparently struggling to breathe. Ferrante was sentenced to life imprisonment in 2015.

Circumstantial Evidence

Because of the secretive nature of poisoning and the fact that there may be no direct witnesses, the prosecution may have to depend on circumstantial evidence more than ideally they would like. Indeed much trail evidence may be circumstantial as Trestrail (2007) points out (Ibid., p. 94).

When baby Terence Armstrong was killed with Seconal sodium, nobody witnessed his father John Armstrong [62] steal the drug. But the fact that a dangerous drugs cupboard had been rifled from the Royal Navy hospital where he worked and among the drugs stolen were 50 Seconal sodium capsules served as indicative evidence. No one directly saw Major Armstrong give arsenic to his wife but the fact that when arrested he was in possession of several individual packets of arsenic was good circumstantial evidence. This was especially so in the light of his unconvincing explanation that he was intending to use the arsenic as weed killer, for if so why carry them as separate packets? As Genene Jones [74] poisoned children in her care, circumstantial evidence was that the rates of expected deaths during her periods of work were much higher than might be expected. Strong circumstantial evidence of motive of greed was revealed in the trial of Frederick Seddon [37] for poisoning his lodger Eliza Barrow as he argued the fine detail of financial transactions with lawyers.

Motive

Naturally, in all homicide trails, not just those involving poisoning, motive will have been discussed by investigators long before the court sits. Like 'intent' motive concerns an internal state and may be difficult to demonstrate convincingly. In the earlier chapter on 'Detection and its avoidance in poison cases', we discussed possible motives for poison homicide. Recall that among possible motives were escaping a relationship, monetary gain, jealousy and sadistic pleasure. A possible motive like driver is 'factitious disorder imposed on another' (American Psychiatric Association 2013, pp. 324–327). An issue at trial is showing convincing evidence of such motives.

If it is to be maintained that *escape from a relationship* is a motive, then evidence that the accused is already having a relationship with someone else other than his or her spouse such as love letters would be relevant. Deep unhappiness with an existing relationship might be shown.

Greed and *monetary gain* may be indicated where the accused accrues wealth from the victim's death, perhaps through inheriting or through life insurance. In several cases, the accused has been shown to have been the one who suggested that the victim take out life insurance. Where there appears to be a pattern of benefitting financially from a death, this can be more convincing as was so with Amy Archer-Gilligan [41] who killed several of her patients to acquire money.

Showing *jealousy* may involve evidence of what the accused said about the object of their jealousy. If the prosecution can set out a situation that could be expected from the accused person's point of view to provoke jealousy this can provide an indication of the possible motive. An example is showing how Jessica Wongso [100] resented the success of her friend Wayan Salihin whom she poisoned at a café in Jakarta, Indonesia with cyanide.

Evidence of *sadistic pleasure* may be suggested by evidence from a diary keeping a record of the suffering of victims. This was the case with Graham Young [68] who killed several work colleagues, taking an intense interest in their sickness and symptoms which he had brought about.

Where the argument is that 'factitious disorder imposed on another' influenced the suspect's behaviour, expert witnesses in psychiatry or psychology may testify. Indications of the suspect's behaviour may contribute to evidence as with the case of Lacey Spears [96] who poisoned her 5-year-old son with sodium (salt) while presenting herself on social media as a devoted mother combatting her son's mysterious illness.

Judge's Summing up and Comments Before Sentence

A judge's summing up of the evidence can be especially influential where a good proportion of evidence may have been technical and therefore hard to assimilate, as well as circumstantial and consequently difficult to evaluate. For example, it has been suggested that the summing up in the trial of Charlotte Bryant [51] for poisoning her husband was detrimental to her and that the depiction of her perceived sexual morals played a part. Such instances are sometimes cited to show that they reflect the values of the time and the expectations about the roles of men and women in society.

Once the verdict has been given, where the accused has been found guilty, the judge may make comments when the perpetrator is sentenced. These may be taken to reflect the views that wider society might hold and are often reported as such by the media. Certain phrases crop up in sentencing comments. The judge may call the poisoner as 'cold and calculating' and refer to the crime as particularly despicable. In 2010, Lakhvir Singh [93] was sentenced to at least 23 years imprisonment for the murder of her lover 'Lucky' Cheema and the grievous bodily harm against his fiancé. Judge Paul Worsley told Singh, 'You were not just a spurned lover; you did not simply explode with anger at the rejection. You set about *a cold and calculating* revenge'. In sentencing the poisoner Angelina Rodriguez [84], Judge William Pounders stated that the murder was 'the coldest killing I have ever seen'. Also, 'Her conduct in administering poison to her husband over a week's time was exceptionally cruel and callous'. The press will often reinforce the calculating nature of the poisoning by noting that the perpetrator 'showed no emotion' as sentence was passed.

Conclusion

Against the background of the legal basis of the crime, at the trial of poisoners, the prosecution seeks essentially to demonstrate proof beyond reasonable doubt in key areas. These are that: the deceased died from poisoning, that the accused administered the fatal dose, and that the accused intended to kill the victim in doing so. Procedures that take place before a trial for poisoning murder are similar to those of other homicide cases.

In trying to show that the deceased died from poisoning it might be suggested that death was owing to natural causes; there may be debate about any indications of poisoning when the victim was dying; and there are likely to be different interpretations of physical evidence that the suspected poison had been administered to the deceased.

When attempting to establish that the accused administered the fatal dose there may be arguments about the relevance or otherwise if the accused was not present when death occurred; whether or not the accused was in possession of the implicated poison; if the accused did possess poison whether they had a legitimate reason; or whether after all death was accidental or caused by suicide.

As the prosecution seeks to demonstrate that the accused both administered the poison and intended to kill the victim it may be argued that although the accused administered the poison there was no intention to kill; or that the accused was insane.

Other issues that can arise at trial include the supposed character of the perpetrator, the role and credibility of witnesses, the use of technical evidence, the extent of circumstantial evidence, and the possible motives of the accused. The judge's summing up and their comments at sentencing may be taken up by the media to convey the particular distaste that society has for homicidal poisoning.

Suggested Activity

According to the legal system pertaining to your country, review the basic procedures for criminal pre-trial and trial (see examples in further reading below) and note the implications where the trial concerns poisoning homicide.

Further Reading

General Criminal Court Procedure

Hemmens, C., Brody, D. C., & Spohn, C. (2017) *Criminal courts: A contemporary perspective* (3rd ed.). Thousand Oaks, CA: Sage.

Sections cover the purpose and structure of US courts, courtroom participants (including the courtroom workgroup), and court processes. Chapter 12 concerns 'The Criminal Trial'.

Sprack, J. (2011). *A practical approach to criminal procedure* (13th ed.). Oxford and New York: Oxford University Press.

This book discusses with great clarity, regarding England and Wales, procedures relating to the Magistrate's Court, the Crown Court, sentencing and appeals.

Particular Poison Trials

For older cases, series such as the 'Notable British Trial Series' are invaluable. For more recent cases, books, book chapters or press court reports may be consulted as indicated in the glossary.

References

American Psychiatric Association. (2013). *Diagnostic and Statistical Manual of Mental Disorders Fifth Edition (DSM5)* Washington DC: APA.

Hemmens, C., Brody, D. C., & Spohn, C. (2017). *Criminal courts: A contemporary perspective* (3rd ed.). Thousand Oaks, CA: Sage.

Loftus, E. (1996). *Eyewitness testimony*. Cambridge, MA: Harvard University Press.

Perry, T., (2008, April and 19). Release of widow ends bizarre case. *Los Angeles Times*.

Sanders, A., & Young, R. (2012). From suspect to trial. In M. Maguire, R. Morgan, & R. Reiner (2012) (Eds.), *The Oxford handbook of criminology* (5th ed.). Oxford: Oxford University Press.

Sprack, J. (2011). *A practical approach to criminal procedure*. Oxford and New York: Oxford University Press.

Trestrail, J. H. (2007). *Criminal poisoning: investigational guide for law enforcement, toxicologists, forensic scientists and attorneys* (2nd ed.). Totowa, NJ: Humana Press.

Chapter 11
Conclusion

Preamble

In aiming to outline criminology of homicidal poisoning, we reviewed theories of crime and homicide in relation to poison murder. We looked at the nature of poisons used in homicides and explored the characteristics of poisoners and their victims and related matters. Discussing aspects of detecting poison homicide, we considered how perpetrators seek to avoid detection. Finally the book raised issues arising when poisoners are brought to trial. Important differences between poison homicide and homicide in general became clear.

Illustrative Poisoning Cases

Examples of cases raising points of special interest: Paul Marshall Curry [95], Julia Lynn Turner [88], Kristin Rossum [82], Roger and David Cooper [99], Dr. Harold Shipman [81], Lakvir Singh [93] and Jessica Wongso [100] illustrate the careful planning that can go into poison homicide but also the meticulous police work that can unravel it. They also point up the 'left of field' nature of some cases. Just when it looks obvious that you plan a poison murder to claim that the deceased died of an accident, suicide or natural causes, a case occurs where the killers dispose of the body. The potential success of revisiting a 'cold case' is shown where the evidence is reinterpreted. We see the length of time that a serial poisoner can go unsuspected and undetected, the danger of sloppy death certification procedures, and the vulnerability of the elderly. Cases reveal police opportunity for detecting a poison murder when the same modus operandi is tried a second time. Motives of perpetrators and the time frames that sometimes confine them become apparent. Also evident is the contribution of some circumstantial evidence in poison cases.

M. Farrell, *Criminology of Homicidal Poisoning*,
DOI 10.1007/978-3-319-59117-9_11

Theories and Explanations

Some poisoning homicides might arise from a 'strain' between society's cultural goals and structural social limitations whether involving financial aspirations or strivings for status and self-reliance. For some poisoners, including serial offenders, delays in the development of their moral reasoning may lead them to succumb to temptation when the opportunity to offend arises. To the extent that a feminist perspective concerns gendered issues, it might shed light on such matters as gender differences between general homicide and poison homicide.

The strongest theme in reviewing theory is the shaping of the offender's behaviour and understanding over time. Rational choice theory (Clarke 1992) concerns factors which influence decisions to commit or desist from criminal activities. For example, individuals can be deterred by controls on the sale and use of poisons and the tightening of death certification procedures. In line with this, where homicide is planned, poisoning is a rational choice because unlike other modus operandi it can more easily allow death to appear to be from natural causes thereby potentially increasing the chances of avoiding detection.

Serial poisoners may be influenced by behavioural reinforcements, social bonds over a considerable period, and through labelling processes. In line with differential reinforcement theory (Jeffrey 1965), serial poisoning and its frequency would be expected to be determined by the positive or negative consequences it creates. Conversant with control theory and related ideas (Laub and Sampson 2003) some serial poisoning may be understood in terms of 'life course' and careers of delinquency in the light of social bonds and other influences over time. According to labelling theory (Becker 1963) the process of labelling may shape the offender's view of themselves and their subsequent behaviour. For example, a serial poisoner may witness media representations and more personal views and reactions (to them their crimes) and gradually shape their offending according to these depictions.

The subcultural theory that the shaping of meaning and the shaping of behaviour itself relates to the mutual mitigation of the crime (e.g. Cohen 1957) might inform explanations of team poisoning.

Understanding Poisons and Their Use in Homicide

Poisons and poisoners can be traced to antiquity and undoubtedly go back to pre-history. Although conceptualising poisons and poisoning is not straightforward, there are accepted definitions. Also, classifications can assist in understanding toxic substances. Certainly, poisons used in homicides in the past and in the present are wide ranging and include: plant, animal and bacterial poisons, drugs, elements their compounds and derivatives, and 'other poisons' such as antifreeze.

This variety and the ubiquitous nature of some poisons such as salt and antifreeze pose challenges for controlling the use of poisons and for detection. For example, lacking odour and taste make certain poisons less detectable. Also, a poisoner's choices are widened by the various routes via which poisons can be administered, and the different ways that they act on the body including mimicking some diseases and illnesses. Such is the nature of poisoning that in comparison with other forms of homicide, it may not even be apparent that any crime has taken place.

Yet such complexities can be reduced by the systematic consideration of poisons such as their characteristics, action, estimated fatal dose, and the treatment of poisoning. The distinction between acute and chronic poisoning can be relevant to understanding the motives of poisoners. Trends suggest that in the past, poisons such as arsenic and cyanide were frequently used while today, narcotics are more commonly detected in poison victims.

Poisoners, Poisoning and General Homicide

Of the poisoner characteristics nominated by Rowland (1960) great ruthlessness seems one of the more convincing especially where the perpetrator administers the substance knowing and witnessing its effects on the victim. Turning to the suggested poisoner traits proposed by Trestrail (2007) the most fitting seem to be cunning, the ability to design and plan in detail, and being (mentally and physically) non-confrontational. Trestrail (2007) in categorising poisoners according to the extent of their planning and the specificity of their victims captures the features of some poisoning cases. Probably the most typical combination of his typology is a poisoner who plans carefully and has a specific victim. The recognition of characteristics such as cunning and planning in detail also reflects what we found in relation to theory where the shaping of behaviour and emotions over time was part of the explanation of poisoning. Again typically a poisoner will arrange matters to make the death appear to be from natural causes as this (all other things being equal) would attract the least suspicion. There are also of course examples where the scenario is made to appear to be suicide or accidental death.

Certain examples of poisoning also reflect motives relating to: money, elimination of someone or something blocking a desired goal, jealousy, revenge, and political motives in one grouping; as well as in another grouping sadism; belief in one's mental superiority, desire to tamper, and boredom-related challenge to law enforcement. None of these characteristics and typologies embraces all poisoners but do illuminate some poisonings.

Marked over-representation of male offenders that typifies general homicides is not reflected in poison homicides. Here there may be still more males than female perpetrators but to nothing like the same extent. Perhaps in the past, female poisoning was commoner than male. If so, it may be because of barriers to divorce for women in unhappy marriages, and the opportunity for women poisoners in their traditional food preparation and caring roles. Peak offender ages for both general and poison homicide appear similar being from late teens to early thirties. Race comparisons between homicide in general and poison homicide do not appear to be possible currently. But for poison killings, offender and victim are usually of the same race. Medical professionals especially but also others whose occupations allow legitimate access to potential poisons are over represented as poisoners. Indeed, one can reasonably speculate that a possible future trend may be an increase in the number of carers found to be involved in poisoning, for example where training, governance and supervision of carers are poor. Those working in domestic or hospitality occupations may also prepare and serve food and drink but are less predominant as perpetrators than medical related poisoners.

Given that the simultaneous poisoning of several victims makes it difficult for the perpetrator to avoid detection, such cases may have several explanations. The poisoner may have not intended to kill, may have meant to kill one person not many, may have a plan to dispose of the bodies, or may have no connection with the victims. Explanations of motives of general serial homicide such as exerting power and control through coercion tend not to apply to poison homicide where such force is not used. Also, whereas serial killing typically alerts the community, medical serial poisoning can long go undetected. Relatedly, offender profiling which can assist the investigation of non-poisoning serial killers is not available with serial poisoners where no one is aware of repeated murder. Regarding team poisoning, subcultural theories of mutually supported mitigation of the crime which relate to general homicide may well also apply. The poisoner's choice of acute or chronic poisoning is likely to reflect particular circumstances for example externally imposed time constraints, or a wish to suggest that the death is owing to a wasting illness. Sometimes, with serial poisoning murder there may be signature features if these can be spotted and the cases connected.

Victims of Poisoning and General Homicide

For homicide in general, victims are highly predominantly male. Regarding homicidal poisoning, male and female victims are either similar in number or there are more male victims, but not in the same degree as for homicides generally. While male-on-male homicides in general are characterised by violent confrontation or revenge, male-on-male poisonings tend to be more considered. Poisoning femicide often of a spouse or lover does not appear motivated by a desire to exert control, as are some non-poisoning femicides, perhaps emerging from a pattern of domestic abuse, although chronic poisoning may be an exception. Female-on-male poisoning tends to involve a spouse or lover. Regarding female-on-female poisonings, recurring motives include romantic or professional jealousy, and financial gain.

Concerning age, in homicide generally, there is a peak range for victims from about 20 to 40 years. For poison homicide victims, some research finds an age peak in the mid to late twenties, while others show peaks for children and the elderly. Where elderly people are murdered for financial gain their selection as victims (given their particular vulnerability and the possibility that death will appear to be from natural causes) will likely involve careful planning and calculation. Relatedly, there may be higher levels of poisoning of elderly people than is currently estimated given that death is often expected and therefore a homicide may go undetected.

For homicide in general, US figure show a higher proportion of black over white victims. It is less clear what the picture is for poison homicides, except that poison victims and offenders are usually of the same race. The social background of poison offenders and victims tends to be similar perhaps reflecting the usually intimate nature of poisoning.

In male-on-male homicides in general often the participants are acquaintances or strangers, but in femicide over a half of women victims are killed by their current or former boyfriend, husband or lover. When women kill, it tends to be intimate partners or ex-partners and family members. For poison victims, the intimate nature of poisoning suggests that there is generally a relationship between poison victim and offender: spouse, lover, relative, friend, co-worker or patient-medic.

The location of many homicides in general is the home and this appears to be similar for poison homicides. Other poisoning venues are nursing homes and hospitals where medics are the perpetrators. Victims have less commonly been poisoned in public places and at their place of work. With poisoning perhaps to a greater extent than with homicides using other weapons, several locations are implicated such as where the poison was obtained, where it was stored, where administered and where discarded.

In looking at individual cases, one can begin to see how the age, gender, race and occupation of the poison victim and offender and the locations involved can interact to influence such features as role expectations and the course of events. A victim's recent contacts, the victim's routines (for example medication regimes) and preferences (such as foods and drinks) and the possible reasons why they became a victim (from the point of view of a suspect) can further add to understanding the crime.

Detection and Its Avoidance in Poisoning Cases

A poisoner can take steps to mask the cause of death of the victim. When a victim is ill, the perpetrator can deflect help or discovery of the symptoms by deterring relatives or friends from visiting. A perpetrator can suggest to the physician attending the victim that what the perpetrator knows is the effect of the poison is really symptoms of illness. When the victim dies, the poisoner may try to avoid autopsy by disguising symptoms as natural causes. They may claim that the deceased objected to autopsy, or if they are the next of kin they may themselves demur. Where it is established that the deceased died of poisoning, the perpetrator may propose an innocent explanation. A crime scene may be arranged by the perpetrator to look as though suicide by poisoning was the cause of death. If the victim had a drug abuse problem, the poisoner might suggest that the cause of death was a self-administered drug overdose by the victim. It may be claimed by the perpetrator that the poison was administered by a third person, deliberately or accidentally. A physician signing a death certificate of someone whom he has killed, or in collusion with an accomplice who has killed, can conceal murder. The murdering physician may exploit the lack of experience of other doctors in getting agreement on death certification, or convince relatives that death had been owing to illness. Sometimes, lack of rigour in the detection process can thwart an arrest.

A wide range of physical evidence can help to prove poisoning. Traces of the poison are clearly potentially incriminating but conversely, an excessively tidy scene may suggest that for example incriminating containers have been cleaned or disposed of. Computer histories may be wiped clean to conceal searches for information about poisons or evidence of ordering poisonous substances on the internet.

A poisoner might attempt avoid the consequences of a later exhumation by pressing for the cremation of the victim if able to do so, although poison traces may be later identified in the cremated ashes. A one-time poisoner using the same modus operandi on a subsequent poisoning has sometimes led to their arrest. Autopsy provides evidence of poisoning both in physical signs and in supplying samples for forensic testing, so if subverted this can frustrate opportunities to gather evidence. Cremation obviously removes the possibility of autopsy. Also, autopsy can be sidestepped by avoiding suspicion for example by setting the scene for an apparently expected death because illness has been previously created by chronic poisoning. Sloppy and corrupted death certification procedures can allow a physician-perpetrator to evade autopsy.

Forensic evidence can be restricted by the poisoner tampering with or destroying potential evidence such bodily fluids excreted when the victim was alive. Any mistake in forensic procedures or communication between departments can allow the poisoner to evade suspicion. Motives for poisoning include: escaping a relationship, monetary gain, jealousy and sadistic pleasure. Motive-like drivers include factitious disorder imposed on another. A constraint which may appear like a motive could be that the perpetrator lacks the physical or emotional characteristics to murder in any other way. Extreme measures can be taken to hide motive including product tampering. Some poisoners through their profession are already knowledgeable about poisons, but where a murder has to gain knowledge of a poison there may be evidence of this. Examples are witnesses to whom the perpetrator spoke, computer files, records of library loans or book purchases. However, the poisoner might: avoid speaking to others of poison, have computer records professionally wiped, or steal or otherwise clandestinely acquire relevant books.

Poisoners need to plan to gain access to noxious substances without leaving a trail. An easily available poison can be stolen, so leaving no record of purchase. Poisons can be made from naturally occurring plants so long as preparations are kept secret. Modern day ability to acquire poisons may be through a person's occupation as with the access of medical personnel to drugs. Poisons can also be obtained from various laboratories. Hobbies can involve using toxic substances. Antique drug and chemical bottles may be misguidedly sold with their contents in place, and of course, poisons can also be stolen.

Opportunity to administer the poison can be disguised. For example, poison can be sent to a victim through the post, although this risks that the wrong person or other people in addition to the victim might consume it. The poisoner may attempt to conceal the poison 'in plain sight'.

Poisoners on Trial

Before the trial, procedures for poisoning murders are similar to those of other homicidal cases. At the trial of poisoners, the prosecution aims to demonstrate proof beyond reasonable doubt in three areas. These are: that the deceased died from poisoning, that the accused administered the fatal dose, and that the accused intended to kill the victim in doing so. While these are the same in essence to what needs to be proved at any homicide trial, the use of poison gives them a distinctive application.

In trying to show that the deceased died from poisoning, the defence team might suggest that death was owing to natural causes; there may be debate about any indications of poisoning when the victim was dying; and there are likely to be different interpretations of physical evidence that the suspected poison had been administered to the deceased.

When attempting to establish that the accused administered the fatal dose there may be arguments about the relevance or otherwise if the accused was not present when death occurred; whether or not the accused was in possession of the implicated poison; or (if the accused did possess poison) whether they had a legitimate reason; or whether after all death was accidental or the result of suicide.

As the prosecution seeks to demonstrate that the accused both administered the poison and intended to kill the victim, defence lawyers may argue that although the accused administered the poison there was no intention to kill; or that the accused was insane.

Other issues that can arise at trial include: the character of the perpetrator, the role and credibility of witnesses, the use of technical evidence, the extent of circumstantial evidence, and the motives of the accused. Of these, perhaps the most distinctive for poison cases is the nature of the technical evidence relating to toxicology for example, and the sometimes extensive reference to circumstantial evidence, given the secretive nature of poison homicide.

The judge's summing up and comments at sentencing are as in all trials important. In poison trials the judge may express particular distaste for the type of murder as being for example 'cold' and 'calculating'. This may be taken up by the media to convey and reinforce the particular abhorrence that society has for homicidal poisoning.

The Poisoner's Position

For someone to poison, sociological and psychological factors may have interacted to prepare the ground for what is to develop. Among these factors which shape behaviour and the meaning of that behaviour are likely to be the most influential, given that poisoning is typically planned and calculated over time. Certain considerations are likely to have arisen for the poisoner. They are in a position where, from their perspective, they consider that drastic action is necessary. Perhaps they face financial pressures or harbour feelings of greed. They may find someone blocking their way to a greatly desired goal, or find someone making their life deeply unfulfilled. For these and other possible reasons, they begin to consider that they can resolve the situation by removing someone that they see as a prime cause or hindrance. Once killing them becomes a possibility, poison is considered as a possible means, more rational than other modes of killing because of the 'extra' possibility that the murder may be made to seem like natural death.

What sort of poison would be suitable? What effect would the poison have? Might it mimic a death by natural causes, or could it be mistaken for symptoms of an illness that the intended victim already has such as epilepsy? Is such a poison available? If so can the prospective poisoner acquire it without leaving a trace of purchase, for example by stealing it? How will it be administered? Will it be injected, given in food or drink or conveyed in some other form?

Let us say the perpetrator now has possession of the poison. Where will it be stored so that it is not found and does not leave traces? When will the poison be given? What routines does the victim follow that could permit this? At which place or places will it be administered? At the victim's work, at home or elsewhere? Would it alleviate any suspicion if the perpetrator were not present when the victim died or might this still draw attention to the killer?

This can be illustrate by many cases but we can outline an example discussed in more detail in the 'Instructive cases' chapter to show the possible thinking. It is that of Lynn Turner's [88] murder of her husband Glenn, the murder that she got away with until she later used the same modus operandi on her common law husband Randy Thompson.

Lynn Turner once she was married to local police officer Glenn Turner left her job and spent lavishly so that her husband took an extra job to keep up with her expenditure. When Glenn started plans to move out and file for a divorce Lynn was already having a secret affair with Randy Thompson, a Forsyth County firefighter. From her viewpoint she saw the prospect of insurance money if her husband died and the chance of moving in with her lover. Killing Glenn would improve matters for her. The timing hinged on her acting before Glenn left and possibly filed for divorce.

The idea of poison may have had the appeal that it was secret and that she might evade detection. Ethylene glycol based antifreeze as a possibility was researched at the local animal shelter. It was accessible and in fact there was a supply in the couple's garage. There would be no need anyways to disguise purchase because it was a legitimate substance so long as poisoning was not suspected. Symptoms might look like natural causes (heart problems).

How would it be administered? Because it is sweet tasting and odourless, many food and drinks could suffice. It is suspected that soup and Jell-O may have been used. The timing and the place where the poison could be administered would be well known to a spouse familiar with her husband's habits and routines. To try to distance herself from the killing Lynn arranged to be out of the house when Glenn died. On her return (so it appeared) she immediately did the right thing when she found Glenn and called for help.

Back to the Issue of Undetected Poisoning

Recall that this planning and foresight allowed Lynn Turner to kill and not be caught the first time round. Other examples where a second offence led to the uncovering on an earlier poisoning undetected at the time are not hard to come by. Catherine Wilson's [10] murder of Maria Soames was only found out when 6 years later the perpetrator was tried and acquitted of attempting to poison another employer and police had the good sense to make wider enquiries. French insurance dealer Henri Girrard [42] poisoned a fellow insurance broker with typhoid bacteria which was unsuspected until 6 years later when he poisoned a certain Mme Monin after insuring her life, making the liable company suspicious. Reverend Frank Sipple [54] poisoned his daughter Dorothy with cyanide but it was 6 years later when the pastor attacked a parishioner that he admitted to the prior crime. In 1978, Marie Hilley [70] tried to poison her daughter and it brought to light the earlier arsenic poisoning of her husband who was thought to have died of infectious hepatitis. When in 1989, Reverend Dwight Moore became ill with suspicious symptoms, police began investigating his wife Blanche Moore [78], eventually establishing that she has poisoned a boyfriend Raymond Reid with arsenic 3 years before.

Other poisoners were unsuspected until an anonymous letter revealed their crime. In France, Dr. Edmund de la Pommerais [11], the homeopathic physician, used digitalis to kill his mistress Seraphine de Pawr but death was deemed to be from natural causes until an unsigned letter soon after her burial led authorities to exhume the body. In England, Dr. Edward Pritchard [12] murdered his wife and his mother-in-law with antimony and aconite declaring on his wife's death certificate that her demise was caused by gastric fever. Both murders were revealed following an unattributed letter to authorities. Lincolnshire dressmaker Ethel Major [49] killed her husband Arthur with strychnine (from a supply kept by her gamekeeper father) the symptoms of which the attending physician thought related to epilepsy until a note to police revealed the true cause.

All these examples leave aside the instances where serial poisoners committing many more murders have gone undetected for years, even decades. Early examples are Mary Bateman [1] and Mary Cotton [14]. Others are Martha Marek [53] of

Vienna, Austria, Nannie Doss [61], in Oklahoma, and Christa Lehman [59] and Anna Zwanziger [2] in Germany. Then there are doctors Marcel Petiot [55], Neill Cream [22], Harold Shipman [81], and Michael Swango [80]; Nurses Orville Lynn Majors [79], and Victorino Chua [98]; nursing aid Donald Harvey [76]; and nursing home managers Arnfinn Nessett [72], Amy Archer-Gilligan [41], and Dorothea Waddingham [50]. Graham Young [68] was detained in a secure psychiatric hospital for poisoning and when released poisoned again. Many others could be cited.

But here, we have come full circle. The suggestion that I made in the 'Introduction' chapter, that poison homicide is likely under estimated, is shown in the vivid light of a real life and all too real death.

References

Becker, H. (1963). *Outsiders.* New York: Free Press.

Clarke, R. V. (Ed.) (1992). *Situational Crime prevention: successful case studies.* New York: Harrow and Heston.

Cohen. A. (1957). *Delinquent boys.* Glencoe: Free Press.

Jeffrey, C. R. (1965). Criminal behaviour and learning theory. *Journal of Criminal Law Criminology and Police Science, 56,* 294–300.

Laub, J., & Sampson, R. (2003). *Shared Beginnings Divergent Lives: Delinquent Boys to Age 70.* Cambridge, Mass: Harvard University Press.

Rowland, J. (1960). *Poisoner in the dock: twelve studies of poisoning.* London: Arco.

Trestrail, J. H. (2007). *Criminal Poisoning: Investigational Guide for Law Enforcement, Toxicologists, Forensic Scientists and Attorneys* (2nd. ed). Totowa, NJ: Humana Press.

Glossary of Poisonings

The list is in chronological order usually of date of sentencing (set in bold) and typically includes:

P Poisoner, year of birth, their country/nationality, occupation where applicable, sentence and date

PA Poison used and how administered

V Victim, their relationship to poisoner, year of their death, venue of murder

M Motive

R Reference for further reading

N Notable other information

1800–1849

[1] P Mary Bateman (née Harker), born 1768, England, confidence trickster, hanged **1809**

PA MB persuaded victim to take a 'protective' concoction (mercuric chloride in honey) for several days, if any ill effects to take an 'antidote' as supplied (arsenic)

V Rebecca Perigo, a gullible acquaintance, died 1806 (Victim's home)

M Financial gain (victim paid for MB's 'protective' services) and to avoid exposure of earlier fraud

R Nash (1981), Davies (2004)

[2] P Anna Zwanziger (née Schönleben), born 1760, Bavaria, Germany, housekeeper, decapitated **1811**

PA Arsenic administered in food and drink while employed as a housekeeper

M. Farrell, *Criminology of Homicidal Poisoning*,
DOI 10.1007/978-3-319-59117-9

V Frau Glaser (wife of Judge Glaser AZ's employer) July 1808, Judge Grohmann (employer) May 1809, Frau Gebhardt (wife of judge Gebhardt AZ's employer) May 1809 (their homes)

M Possibly a sense of power over victims

R Emsley (2005)

[3] P Dr. Edme Castaing, born 1796, France, physician, guillotined **1823**

PA Morphine acetate powder in wine and in a medicinal draught

V Hippolyte Ballet, fellow conspirator in forging the Will of Ballet's brother Auguste, 1823 (victim's home)

M Financial gain from victim's Will

R Parry (1927)

[4] P Marie Lafarge, born 1816, France, sentenced to life imprisonment **1840**, released with ill-health 1852 and died same year

PA Arsenic in eggnog, possibly earlier in cake, venison, and truffles

V Charles Pouch-Lafarge, her husband, 1840 (at the Lafarge home)

M Disillusionment with her husband, the (false) expectation to inherit from his Will

R Saunders, 1951

[5] P John Tawell, born 1784, Berkshire, England, chemist, hanged **1845**

PA Prussic acid added to a bottle of 'stout' (beer)

V Sarah Lawrence (later changed to Hart), his mistress, 1845 (at her house)

M A married man and a Quaker, JT feared exposure of the clandestine relationship with his mistress

R Farrell (1992)

1850–1899

[6] P Count Hippolyte de Bocarmé, born 1818, Mons, Belgium, aristocrat, guillotined **1851**

PA Distilled nicotine administered forcibly by mouth

V His brother-in-law Gustave Fougnies, 1851 (Count's chateau where he was a dinner guest)

M Financial gain

R Farrell (1992)

[7] P Hélèna Jégado, born 1803, Brittany, France, domestic servant, guillotined **1852**

PA Administered in food and drink

V Perotte Mace, fellow worker at Bout-du-Monde Hotel, Rennes, 1850 (at the hotel); Rose Tessier, 1850; Rosalie Sarrazin, 1851, both fellow servants for Theophile Bidard a law professor in Rennes (at their workplace Bidard's home)

M Jealousy

R Heppenstall (1970)

N At trial HJ was accused of three murders, three attempted murders and various thefts, and was highly suspected of many other murders

[8] P Dr. William Palmer, born 1824, Rugeley, England, physician, hanged **1856**

PA Strychnine in pills given as supposed medication

V Companion John Cook, 1856 (at the Talbot Arms Hotel, Rugeley where Cooke was staying)

M Financial gain

R Watson (1856/1952), St. Aubyn (1971)

[9] P Dr. William King, born c1830, Canada, teacher and homoeopathic physician, hanged **1859**

PA Arsenic probably in food and drink

V His wife Sarah, 1859 (at their home in Brighton, Ontario)

M To be with Melinda Vandervoort with whom he was infatuated

R Dougal (2016)

[10] P Wilson, born 1822, Lincolnshire, England, live-in nurse, hanged **1862**

PA Colchicum probably in food

V Maria Soames, killed in London 1856, (the victim's home where CW was a lodger)

M Probably monetary gain

R Farrell (1992)

N Murder of 1856 undiscovered until 1862 when CW was tried and acquitted of attempting to poison a woman employer and police enquiries uncovered the earlier death. CW was also suspected of other poison murders.

[11] P Dr. Edmund de la Pommerais, born 1846, France, homoeopathic physician, Guillotined **1864**

PA Digitalis, unclear how administered.

V His mistress a widow Seraphine de Pawr (1863) (at her home in Paris)

M Financial gain from an insurance policy on de Pawr's life

R Thorwald (1966)

N Death deemed natural causes until an anonymous letter soon after burial led authorities to exhume the body

[12] P Dr. Edward Pritchard, born 1825, Hampshire, England, physician, hanged **1865**

PA Antimony (and aconite) at their home in Glasgow, Scotland. For Jane Tailor (mother in law) in the opiate medicine Battley's Solution. For Mary Jane Cowan (wife) in food

V Jane Tailor aged 70 years who was nursing her ill daughter, February 1865; and Mary Jane Cowan, March, 1865, both revealed following anonymous letter to authorities

M Possibly to allow continuation of an affair with a housemaid

R Roughhead (1906)

N Dr. James Patterson declined to sign the death certificates. Pritchard signed them himself (wife, gastric fever). Wife's 'illness' abated when she stayed with her mother Christmas 1864, but resumed when she returned to husband

[13] P Marie Jeanneret, born 1836, Switzerland, nurse, sentenced to 20 years imprisonment **1868**, died 1884

PA Belladonna (and other poisons) administered as medicines

V Charged with killing: Douise Junod, Jeanne Gray, Jenny Juvet, Louise Henriette, Mme. Bourcart, Jaques Gros, Julie Bonvier, Mme. Legeret, Demoiselle Fritzges. Convicted of killing seven patients

M Probably sadistic

R *New York Times*, 11 May, 1884

[14] P Mary Ann Cotton née Robson, born 1832, Sunderland, England, housekeeper/nurse/dressmaker, hanged **1873**

PA Arsenic possibly administered with arrowroot which MAC admitted using for son's illness

V Charles Edward Cotton, her son, 1873

M To be rid of her son to enable her to take a job as a nurse

R Appleton (1973)

N Highly suspected of poisoning previous husbands and lovers for financial gain and generally regarded as a serial killer

[15] P Pierre Désiré Moreau, born 1842, Paris, herbalist, guillotined **1874**

PA Copper sulphate (found in both exhumed bodies) unclear how administered

V Wife Félicye-hortense Aubry, 1869; Second wife, Adelaide-Louise (Lagneau) 1874, both at home

M Financial gain

R *Quotidien Le Gaulois*, 11 September 1874

[16] P Eugène Chantrelle, born 1834, Nantes, France, school teacher, hanged **1878**

PA Opium in fruit drinks

V His wife Elizabeth Dyer, 1878, at their home, Edinburgh, Scotland

M Financial gain from life insurance

R Smith (1906)

N Attempted to present death as accidental poisoning from a damaged gas main

[17] P Dr. George Lamson, born 1850, England; physician; hanged **1882**

PA Aconite in slice of shared Dundee cake

V Percy John his 18-year-old brother-in-law, 1881; at PJ's boarding school, Wimbledon, England

M Financial gain

R Browne and Stewart ([1883]/2015), St. Aubyn (1971)

[18] P Louisa Taylor, born about 1848, London, milliner and widow of HM Customs worker, Hanged **1883**

PA 'Sugar of lead' administered in medicine

V Her friend (aged in her eighties) Mary Ann Tregillis at whose house she had been staying for several weeks after being widowed, 1882

M Financial gain, Mr. Tregillis reported that LT had stolen and sold items from his home

R Emsley (2005)

[19] P Israel Lipski (previously Lobulsk), born 1865, London, Umbrella/walking stick maker, hanged **1887**

PA Nitric acid administered forcibly by mouth

V Miriam Angel a married woman, 1887 (in her bedroom at the lodging house, London where IL was also a tenant)

M Prosecution claimed in relation to attempted rape, IL claimed robbery

R Friedland (1984)

N IL was discovered hiding under Miriam's bed, acid burns around his mouth

[20] P Dr. Philip Cross, born 1825, Ireland, physician, hanged **1888**

PA Arsenic probably added to Laura's sodium bromide medication

V His wife Laura, 1887, (at their home Shandy Hall)

M To marry his lover Effie Skinner, 43 years his junior, and previously his children's governess

R Duke (1934)

N Dr. Cross 'diagnosed' his wife's poisoning symptoms as typhoid, certifying her death accordingly

[21] P Florence Maybrick née Chandler, born 1862, Alabama, wife of an English cotton broker, Imprisoned **1889**, released 1904, died in US 1941

PA Arsenic (which James also took medicinally) possibly with other medicines

V Her husband James, 1889 (at their home in Liverpool, England)

M Unhappy marriage, both she and husband had lovers. He had threatened divorce

R Irving (1912)

[22] P Dr. Neill Cream, born 1850, Glasgow (Lived Canada, US, and London), physician, hanged **1892**

PA Strychnine including in drinks

V Four prostitutes: Helen Donworth (Oct 1891), Matilda Clover (October 1891), Emma Showell, and Alice Marsh jointly murdered (April 1892) at various venues

M Probably sadistic although he did not remain to witness the deaths of his victims, possibly hoped for monetary gain from extortion.

R Farrell (1993a, b)

N In 1881 Cream imprisoned in Illinois for poisoning Daniel Scott with strychnine. Released 1891. London murders, attracted attention by sending accusatory letters fictitiously implicating others and demanding money

[23] P Dr. Etienne Deschamps, born 1830, France, Dentist, hanged **1892**

PA Chloroform which was also used on previous occasions to make the victim unconsciousness

V 12-year-old Juliette Deitsh, 1892 (at his New Orleans practice offices)

M ED convinced victim's father that Juliette as an occult source helping ED to detect lost treasure and sexually abused her

R Tallant (1953)

[24] P Carlysle Harris, born 1868, New York, medical student, electrocuted **1893**

PA Morphine overdose introduced into medication for insomnia which CH had (illegally) prescribed

V Mary Helen Potts to whom he was secretly 'married' in 1890 under assumed names, murdered 1891, (At her boarding school, New York)

M Possibly to avoid a legitimate church wedding demanded by Mary's mother

R Boswell and Thompson (1961)

[25] P Dr. Robert Buchanan, born 1860, Nova Scotia, Physician, electrocuted **1895**

PA Morphine, probably administered in spoonful of supposed medicine

V His second wife Anna née Sutherland, brothel keeper, 1885 (at their New York home)

M Financial gain from inheritance

R Farrell (1992)

N Soon after killing his second wife, RB discretely remarried his first wife Helen.

[26] P Edith Carew, born 1868, Glastonbury, England, wife of Walter Carew a club secretary, sentenced to death **1897**, commuted to penal servitude for life, ultimately served in England, released 1910, died 1968

PA Arsenic possibly administered with food or medicine

V Her husband Walter, 1896, Yokohama, Japan

M Possibly to rekindle an affair with a lover Dickinson which he had recently terminated.

R Whittington-Egan (2012)

[27] P Walter Horsford, born 1870, Spaldwick, Cambridgeshire, England, farmer, hanged **1898**

PA Strychnine posted by WH with instructions to take it. Victim believed would induce abortion

V His cousin the widow Annie Holmes pregnant with his child, 1898 (at her home in St. Neots, Cambridgeshire)

M To avoid the embarrassment of an illegitimate child

R Farrell (1993a)

[28] P Cordelia Botkin, born 1854, Missouri, US, sentenced life imprisonment **1898**, died in prison 1910

PA Arsenic in chocolates sent by post from San Francisco where CB lived to victim in Dover, Delaware

V Her lover's estranged wife, Mary Dunning, and Mary's sister Ida Harriet Deane, 1898 (at victim's home in Delaware)

M Jealous belief that her lover John Dunning who had left his wife to live with CB might return to his wife

R Rodell (1947)

1900–1949

[29] P George Chapman (Severin Klosowski), born 1865, Poland, publican, hanged **1903**

PA Antimony

V His lover Maud Marsh, barmaid, 1902 (at their residence in London)

M Unclear

R Adam (1930)

N Highly suspected of also poisoning two former lovers

[30] P Sarah Anne Pearson and Agnes Black (neé Pearson), both wives of labourers, County Armagh, Ireland, sentenced to hanging **1904**, commuted to penal servitude for life 1905

PA Strychnine probably administered with food

V Alice Pearson aged 74, retired domestic servant, (Agnes' mother and Sarah's mother in law) 1905

M Financial gain

R Farrell (1992)

[31] P Arthur Deveureux, born 1881, London, chemist's assistant, hanged **1905**

PA Morphine purporting to be cough medicine administered to all three victims

V His wife Beatrice and twin 2-year-old sons Laurence and Evelyn, 1905

M To better provide for his remaining (and favourite) son Stanley

R Browne and Tullett (1951)

N Disposed of the three bodies in a warehouse**??**

[32] P 'Johan Hoch' (born John Schmidt), born Germany, 1855, emigrated to US, meat packer, hanged **1906**

PA Arsenic, unclear how administered

V His wife Julia Walcker-Hoch, 1906 (at their Chicago home)

M Expediency, soon after the killing he married his new sister in law whom he quickly deserted taking some of her money

R Smith (1923)

N Suspected of killing for financial gain other women whom he bigamously married

[33] P Richard Brinkley, born 1853, London, carpenter, hanged **1907**

PA Prussic acid in a bottle of stout (beer)

V Intending to kill a potential witness to forgery Reginald Parker, instead killed Parker's visiting landlord and wife Richard and Elizabeth Beck, 1907 (Parker's house)

M Intention to kill potential witness to forgery

R Oddie (1941)

[34] P Martha Rendell, Perth, Australia, hanged **1909**

PA Hydrochloric acid as a mouth swab for supposed sore throat

V Her step son Arthur Morris (14) in 1908

M Sadistic

R Skehan, date unknown

N Suspected of killing step daughters Annie Morris (aged 7) and Olive Morris (5) 1907 and 1908

[35] P Dr. Hawley Harvey Crippen, born 1862, Michigan, US, later moved to England, hanged **1910**

PA Hyoscine, administration unclear

V His second wife Cora Turner (Kunigunde Mackamotski), 1910 (at their London home)

M To be with his lover Ethel le Neve

R Young (1950), Foran et al. (2011)

N Police found remains buried in in cellar of London home considered to be those of Cora. With the aid of wireless communication, Crippen and le Neve arrested fleeing for Canada on SS Montrose. DNA reported in 2011 testing of a sample of tissue raised questions about the identity of the remains.

[36] P Adolph Hofrichter, born 1880, Bohemia, officer in infantry regiment, sentenced to imprisonment **1910**, pardoned 1919.

PA Potassium cyanide capsules posted to several officers as supposed aphrodisiacs from a pharmacist

V Captain Richard Mader, 1909

M Jealousy at the promotion of fellow officers

R Fahey (2011)

[37] P Frederick Seddon, born 1870, Liverpool, Later moved to London, Insurance superintendent, hanged **1911**

PA Arsenic probably extracted from fly papers, possibly administered in tonics

V Eliza Barrow, 1911 (at FS home where she was a lodger)

M Financial gain

R Young ([1914]/1952)

[38] P Reverend Clarence Richeson, born 1876, Virginia, US, Baptist minister, electrocuted **1912**

PA Potassium cyanide given as supposed medicine

V Girlfriend Avis Linnell, who was pregnant with his child, 1911 (at YMCA student boarding house, Boston)

M Engaged to another woman, CR wanted to avoid Avis Linnell's pregnancy becoming known

R Farrell (1992)

[39] P Augusta Fullam, born 1875, England, later lived in colonial India, sentenced to death **1913**, commuted to penal servitude for life, died of heatstroke 1914. Dr. Henry Clark, born 1868, India, physician, hanged **1913**

PA Arsenic in his Sanatogen tonic and food

V Augusta's husband Edward McKean Fullam, 1911 (At his home in Agra, India)

M Double murder of their spouses to be able to marry each other

R Farrell (1992)

N Also procured the murder of Louisa Clarke (Henry Clarke's wife) by sword, 1912

[40] P Dr. Arthur Waite, born 1889, US, dentist, electrocuted **1917**

PA Diphtheria and tuberculosis germs (and arsenic)

V Hannah Peck and John Peck his parents-in-law, 1917 (Waite's Grand Rapids, NY apartment)

M Financial gain from inheritance

R Buhk (2014)

[41] P Amy Archer-Gilligan (née Duggan), born c1868, possibly Connecticut, sentenced to death **1917**, granted new trial and pleaded guilty to second-degree murder, sentenced to life imprisonment 1919, certified insane 1934, died 1962.

PA Arsenic unclear how administered

V Franklin Andrews, former resident of her Connecticut Nursing Home

M Financial gain

R Phelps (2010)

N Highly suspected of killing Michael Gilligan (her second husband) and Amy Hosmer, Alice Gowdy and one other person who were previous residents of her nursing home

[42] P Henri Girrard, born 1875, France, insurance dealer, committed suicide awaiting trial **1921**

PA Typhoid bacteria from a scientific suppliers, injected as supposed camphorated camomile

V Louis Pernotte an insurance broker, 1912, at Pernotte's Paris home

M Financial gain from life insurance

R Kershaw (1974)

N The murder went unsuspected until in 1918 HG apparently poisoned a Mme Monin after insuring her life and following insurance company suspicions he was arrested

[43] P Major Herbert Armstrong, born 1869, Devon, solicitor, hanged **1922**

PA Arsenic probably administered in food and drink

V Wife Katherine, 1922, at their home Hay on Wye (Welsh English border)

M To be rid of dominating wife, sexual freedom

R Young (1927), Farrell (1989b)

[44] P Edward Black, born 1885, Cornwall, England, insurance seller, hanged **1922**

PA Arsenic unclear how administered

V His wife Annie, sweet shop owner, 1922

M unclear

R Farrell (1992)

N EB away from home when wife died but was traced to Liverpool

[45] P Jean Pierre Vaquier, born 1879, France, lecturer in radio, hanged **1924**

PA Strychnine in Alfred Jones' health salts

V Alfred Jones, proprietor of the hotel and husband of JPVs lover Mabel Jones 1924 (Blue Anchor Hotel, Surrey, England)

M To be with his lover whom he had met on holiday in Biarritz

R Blundell and Seaton (1929)

[46] P Daisy de Melker, Born 1886, Cape Province, South Africa, nurse, hanged **1932**

PA Arsenic in flask of coffee

V Her son, Rhodes Cowle aged 20 years, 1932

M Unclear but apparent abhorrence of son

R Bennett (1974, 1993a)

N Tried but acquitted of the strychnine poisoning of previous husbands William Cowle, 1923, and Robert Sproat, 1927

[47] P Dan Keisberg, Tony Marino, Joseph Murphy, Francis Pasqua, (all electrocuted **1933**), Hershey Green (sentenced to imprisonment **1933**)

PA Carbon monoxide gas (Murphy's room, New York City)

V Mike Malloy, a vagrant, 1933

M Financial gain from life insurance

R Read (2005)

N Several previous attempts on victim's life had failed

[48] P Reginald Hinks, born 1900, England, vacuum cleaner seller, hanged **1934**

PA Carbon monoxide (in coal gas) which RH claimed was owing to suicide

V James Pullen his father-in-law, aged 85 years, 1933 (house in Bath, England shared with his daughter)

M To gain sole use of the house where RH lived with his wife and the victim

R Rowland, 1957

[49] P Ethel Major, born 1892, Lincolnshire, England, dressmaker, hanged **1934**

PA Strychnine (from a supply kept by her gamekeeper father for vermin) added to corned beef

V Her husband Arthur 1934

M Marital estrangement

R Bowker, 1947

N Attending physician thought symptoms related to epilepsy. Crime revealed by an anonymous note to police

[50] P Dorothea Waddingham, born 1899, Hucknall, Nottinghamshire, England, nursing home manager, hanged **1936**

PA Overdose of morphine tablets

V Louisa Baguley (aged 89) May 1935, and her daughter Ada Baguley (aged 50) September 1935 (both at DW's nursing home, Nottingham, England)

M Financial gain from inheritance made over in exchange for the patients' care

R Glaister (1954)

N DW claimed untruthfully that Dr. Mansfield had given her surplus morphine tablets for Ada Baguley

[51] P Charlotte Bryant (née McHugh), England, hanged **1936**

PA Arsenical weed killer in Oxo drink

V Husband Frederick, farm labourer recently made unemployed, 1935 (at their home in Coombe, Somerset, England)

M To be solely with her lover Leonard Parsons a pedlar who lodged at the Bryant's cottage

R Farrell (1989a, 1990)

N CB had previous affairs, apparently tolerated by her husband, which seems to have gone against her in court

[52] P Mary Creighton born 1898, housewife, and Everett Applegate, born 1899, New York State, US, both electrocuted **1936**

PA Arsenical rat poison in milk

V Everett's wife Ada Applegate, September 1936 (the Creighton's home, Baldwin, New York)

M Possibly arising from sexual relationships apparently existing between the two families

R Farrell (1992)

N Everett and Ada Applegate moved in with their neighbours John and Mary Creighton to save money during the Great Depression. MC had previously twice been tried and acquitted of murder by poisoning and police linked Ada Applegate's death with these.

[53] P Martha Marek (née Lowenstein) born 1904, Vienna, Austria; guillotined **1938**

PA Thallium bought from a pharmacist in Vienna probably administered in food

V Her husband Emil Marek (July 1932), her daughter Ingeborg (August 1932), a relative Susanne Lowenstein (July 1934), and a lodger Frau Kittenberger, 1937

M Financial gain from life insurance and inheritance

R Emsley (2005), pp. 332–333

N Frau Kittenberger's son suspecting MM persuaded authorities to exhume his mother's body in which thallium was found. Previous victims' bodies were then exhumed and thallium found.

[54] P Reverend Frank Sipple, born (date unknown), US, pastor, sentenced to life imprisonment **1946**, released in late 1959 on health grounds, died early 1960.

PA Cyanide capsule, possibly given as a medication or in food

V His 18-year-old daughter Dorothy Ann Sipple, 1939, (at the family home Grand Rapids, Michigan)

M FS claimed that his daughter was mentally disturbed and better dead.

R Trestrail (2007), pp. 15–16.

N Homicide undiscovered until 1946 when after attacking a parishioner, FS admitted to killing Dorothy Ann

[55] P Dr. Marcel Petiot, born 1897, Auxerre, France, physician, guillotined **1946**

PA Cyanide injections purporting to be vaccinations for victims' country of destination

V 24 men and women 1942–1944 during Nazi occupation of France (at his Paris home)

M Financial gain from payment for 'escape' and robbery of victims' valuables

R Maeder (1980)

N Victims lured to his surgery with the promise of a safe passage to an unoccupied country, poisoned then bodied burned. MP claimed to work for French Resistance and that the deceased were Nazi collaborators.

1950–1999

[56] P Sadamichi Hirasawa, born 1892, Japan, artist (painter), sentenced to death **1950**, following legal argument this changed to life imprisonment, died in prison 1987

PA Cyanide drink, which SH posing as an official, told employees was a dysentery inoculation

V Twelve members of bank staff, 1948 (at a Tokyo bank)

M Financial gain from bank robbery

R Morikawa (1977)

[57] P Teresa Miriam Conroy, born 1909, London, found guilty but insane, **1953**, detained indefinitely

PA Carbon-monoxide gas and methylphenobarbitone

V Her 13-year-old son, 1953 (at their home in London)

M Court judged insanity

R Farrell (1992)

N TC hid her son's body in a mattress then went away for several days. The corpse was soon after discovered by her husband John Conroy

[58] P Louisa Merrifield, born 1906, England, housekeeper, hanged **1953**

PA Rat poison containing phosphorus

V Her employer as housekeeper 79-year-old Sarah Anne Ricketts, 1953 (at Rickett's home Blackpool, England)

M Financial gain through inheritance

R Wilson (1971)

[59] P Christa Lehman (née Ambrose), born 1922, Worms, Germany, life imprisonment **1954**

PA E605 administered to her husband Karl in milk, to Valentin Lehman in yoghurt, to Annie Hamann in candies/sweets

V Her husband Karl, 1942, and Valentin Lehman her father-in-law 1952, her friend Annie Hamann 1954

M Unclear, poisoning of Annie Hamann was inadvertent

R Farrell (1992)

[60] P Arthur Ford, born 1910 London, chemical company office manager, sentenced to five years imprisonment for manslaughter **1954**

PA Cantharides in sweets/candies

V June Malins and Betty Grant (work secretaries)

M To sexually arouse a secretary to whom he was attracted thinking cantharides was an aphrodisiac

R Farrell (1992)

[61] P Nannie Doss, born 1905, Aniston, Alabama, sentenced to life imprisonment **1955**, died 1965

PA Arsenic administered in food and drink

V Her mother, sister Dovie, grandson Robert, the mother of one of her five husbands Arlie Laning, and four husbands 1920s-1954 (Alabama, Oklahoma, Kansas, North Carolina)

M Financial gain from insurance, although ND claimed boredom

R Trestrail (2007), p. 18.

[62] P John Armstrong, born 1930, England, sick berth attendant at a naval hospital, sentenced to death **1956**, commuted to imprisonment.

PA Seconal sodium in capsules

V His baby son Terence aged 5 months, 1955

M Unclear

R Farrell (1995)

[63] P Kenneth Barlow, born 1919, England, nurse, sentenced life imprisonment **1958**, released 1984

PA Insulin injection before drowning

V His second wife Elizabeth, 1957 (bathroom of their home in Bradford, Yorkshire, England)

M Possibly marital strains, wife was pregnant

R Farrell (1995)

N Arranged scene to suggest accidental drowning

[64] P Mary Wilson, born 1893, South Tyneside, England, sentenced to death **1958**, commuted to life imprisonment, died in prison 1962

PA Phosphorus beetle poison, possibly administered with medication

V Oliver Leonard retired estate agent/realtor, aged 75 (second husband) killed 1956, Ernest Wilson, retired engineer, aged 76 (third husband) killed 1957 (home in Gateshead, Tyne-and-Wear, England)

M Financial gain from money and property

R Farrell (1994)

N Suspected of murdering John Knowles (first husband) and John Russell (her lover)

[65] P Master Sergeant Marcus Marymont, born 1921, US, later stationed at US air base in Norfolk, England, sentenced to life imprisonment **1958** by US General Court Martial, returned to Kansas, US to serve sentence

PA Arsenic administered the day before victim's collapse probably in food

V His wife Mary Helen Marymont, 1958, (collapsed at a luncheon in Kings Lynn, Norfolk, England, later died in hospital)

M Was having a relationship with another woman

R Emsley (2005)

[66] P Dr. Carl Coppolino, born 1933, US, former anaesthetist, sentenced to life imprisonment **1967** for second-degree murder, paroled 1979

PA Succinylcholine chloride (an anaesthetic) as an injection overdose

V His wife Dr. Carmela Musetto, 1967 (at their home in Florida)

M To be able to marry lover

R Holmes (1968)

[67] P Maria Groesbeek, (née Deysel) born 1936, North West Province, South Africa, hanged **1970**

PA Arsenical ant poison administered in food

V Her husband Christian Buys 1969

M Revenge for husband's refusal of divorce. Ten weeks after victim's death she married lover Gerhard Groesbeek

R Bennett (1974)

[68] P Graham Young, born 1947, London, England, store worker at a photographic suppliers, sentenced to life imprisonment **1972**, died in prison 1990

PA Thallium, administered in tea which he made for co-workers. GY kept a diary of the doses and effects of his poisonings.

V Work colleagues Bob Egle 1971 and Fred Biggs, 1971 (both became ill at work, died in hospital)

M Sadism, obsession

R Emsley (2005)

N In 1962, aged 15, GY admitted to Broadmoor secure psychiatric hospital, confessing to administering poison to his father a sister and a school friend. He was released in 1970.

[69] P Steven Roy Harper, born 1955, Omaha, Nebraska, US, researcher at Eppley Research Institute, Omaha, sentenced to death **1979**, committed suicide awaiting penalty

PA *N*-Nitrosodimethylamine in lemonade and milk

V Duane Johnson aged 24, and 11-month-old Chad, the husband and baby respectively of Sandra Johnson, Harper's former girlfriend, 1978 (at the Johnson home)

M Jealousy

R Roueche (1982)

[70] P Marie Hilley, born 1933, US, arrested 1979, escaped, sentenced in absentia for husband's murder **1980**, fugitive until 1983, incarcerated, escaped 1987, died of hyperthermia

PA Arsenic, unclear how administered

V Her husband Frank Hilley, 1975, (Anniston, Alabama, US)

M Financial gain from insurance

R McDonald (1986)

N Attempted to poison daughter in 1978, bringing to light earlier murder of husband whom it was thought died of infectious hepatitis.

[71] P Susan Barber, born 1953, Essex, England, wife of factory worker, sentenced to life imprisonment **1982**

PA Paraquat in food

V Her husband Michael, 1982 (at home Westclife-on-sea, Essex, England, died in hospital)

M Revenge. Victim had beaten SB and her lover Richard Collins after finding them naked together at his home

R Wilson and Seaman (1983)

[72] P Arnfinn Nessett, born in Trǿndelag, Norway, 1936, nurse, sentenced to imprisonment **1983**, released 2004

PA Succinylcholine chloride administered as supposed medication

V 21 residents of his nursing home in Orkdallo, Norway, 1977–1980

M Possibly feelings of power

R Wilson and Seaman (1983)

[73] P Ronald Clark O'Bryan, born 1944, Pasadena, Texas, optician, executed by lethal injection, **1984**

PA Potassium cyanide administered in candy

V Timothy his 8-year-old son, 1974 Texas

M Financial gain from life insurance

R Trestrail (2007), pp. 19–20.

[74] P Genene Jones, born 1950, Texas, US, paediatric nurse, sentenced to extensive prison sentences **1984**

PA Succinylcholine and other drugs by injection

V 15-month-old Chelsea McClellan, another child Rolando Santos, suspected of killing many more children, (at various medical clinics, San Antonio, Texas) 19777–1982

M Endangered children's lives then sought adulation by 'saving' them

R Hickey (2010)

[75] P Stella Nickell, née Stephenson, born 1943, Oregon, US, sentenced to 99 years imprisonment **1987**

PA Cyanide, added to Excedrin capsules

V Husband Bruce Nickell, Susan Snow a bank manager, 1986 (Auburn, Washington)

M Financial gain from insurance

R Trestrail (2007), pp. 22–23

N Poisoned husband then replaced shop stock with poisoned capsules ('product tampering') killing Susan Snow randomly

[76] P Donald Harvey, born 1952, Ohio, hospital worker, sentenced to life imprisonment **1987**

PA Cyanide and other poisons and methods

V DH pleaded guilty to 24 killings, mainly patients at hospitals in Kentucky and Ohio, between 1970 and 1987

M Compulsive serial killer, claimed to be easing patients' suffering

R Trestrail (2007), p. 23

[77] P George Trepal, born 1949, Florida, US, former chemist, sentenced to death **1991**

PA Thallium added to bottles of 'Coca-Cola'

V Neighbour Peggy Carr, 1988 (Polk County, Florida)

M Revenge following several altercations

R Trestrail (2007), pp. 23–24.

[78] P Blanche Moore (nee Kiser), born 1933, North Carolina US, sentenced to death **1991**, still awaiting penalty 2016

PA Arsenic administered in food

V Her boyfriend Raymond Reid, 1986

M Apparent hatred of men following maltreatment by her father

R *Washington Times*, 2015

N Suspected of poisoning father P. D. Kiser (1968), mother in law Isla Taylor (1970), and first husband James Taylor (1971). Police began investigating after BM's second husband Rev Dwight Moore developed suspicious symptoms in 1989

[79] P Orville Lynn Majors, born 1961, Indiana, US, nurse, sentenced to 360 years imprisonment **1999**

PA Potassium chloride and epinephrine

V Patients at Vermillion County Hospital 1993–1994: Mary Anderson 69, Dorothea Hixon, 80, Cecil Smith, 74, Luella Hopkins, 89, Margaret Hornick, 79, Freddie Wilson, 56, Derek Maxwell, 64

M Hated elderly people

R Hanna (1999)

2000–2017

[80] P Dr. Michael Swango, born 1954, Tacoma, Washington, US, physician, arrested 1997, sentenced to life imprisonment **2000**

PA Arsenic added to food and drink

V 4 patients (may have been many more between 1981 and 1997)

M Unclear

R Stewart (1999)

[81] P Dr Harold Shipman, born 1946, Nottingham, England, physician, sentenced to life imprisonment **2000**, committed suicide in prison 2004

PA Mainly morphine based drugs

V 250 of his patients 1970 to 1990s (Yorkshire and Manchester, England often in their own homes)

M Possibly feelings of power over life and death

R Peters (2005)

N Convicted of 15 murders, a subsequent public enquiry established that he was responsible for about 250

[82] P Kristin Rossum, born 1976, Claremont, California, US, former toxicologist, sentenced to life imprisonment **2002**

PA Fentanyl, stolen from her workplace at Medical Examiner's Office

V Husband Greg de Villers, worked at a biotech company, 2000 (San Diego)

M Husband discovered KR having an affair with her boss Michael Robertson, and taking illegal drugs, and threatened to reveal this unless she quit her job

R Glatt (2004); www.legacy.sandiegouniontribune.com/news/metro/rossum/

N KR arranged scene to look like suicide

[83] P Daniel Bondeson, born 1950, US, potato farmer, suicide leaving a confessional note, 5 days after killing, **2003**

PA Arsenic possibly obtained from old farm chemical products added to congregation's coffee after church service

V Walter Morrill aged 78, a fellow church worshiper, 2003 (in Lutheran Church Portland, Maine)

M Following internal disputes at the Church

R Davy (2003)

N Also made15 other church members ill.

[84] P Angelina Rodriguez, born 1968, Queens, New York, US, sentenced to death **2004**

PA Ethylene glycol based antifreeze in Gatorade

V Her fourth husband Frank Rodriguez, a special education teacher, 2000 (at their home, Montebello, Los Angeles County)

M Financial gain from insurance

R Gorman (2004)

[85] P Daisuke Mori, born 1971, Japan, nurse, arrested 2001, sentenced to life imprisonment **2004**

PA Vecuronium bromide overdose

V Yukiko Shimoyama 89-year-old woman 2000 (at clinic in Izumi-ku, Sendai, Japan)

M Unclear

R Author uncredited, 2004 *The Japan Times* 31 March

N Suspected of four attempted murders of patients in 2000. Hospital also criticised.

[86] P Ryan Furlough, born 1987, US, high school student, sentenced to life imprisonment **2004**

PA Cyanide (bought via internet) administered in soda drink

V His friend Benjamin Vassilev, aged 17 years, 2003, (basement of RF home, Ellicott City, Baltimore, US)

M Jealousy over Vassilev's girlfriend, RF felt his friend no longer cared for him,

R Trestrail (2007), p. 25.

[87] P Wei Entan, born 1977, Nanjiang, Pingjiang County, China, farmer, attempted suicide hours after the poisoning in 2003, sentence was expected 2004 but unknown

PA 'Dushuquaing' or 'strong rat poison' (tetramethyenedisulfotetramine), administered in fruit

V Yu Yuanfang Chen and Yu Xuling Chen, son and daughter of his married lover (at their elementary school) 2003

M Revenge over affair with married lover ending

R Hoo (2003)

[88] P Lynn Turner (born Julia Lynn Womack), born 1968, Texas, US, 911 dispatcher, sentenced to imprisonment **2004** (and 2007), committed suicide in prison 2010

PA Ethylene glycol antifreeze in food

V Former husband police officer Glenn Turner 1995 (for which sentenced in 2004) and boyfriend fire officer Randy Thompson 2002 (for which sentenced 2007)

M Financial gain

R Martinez (2010)

N Death of Randy Thompson alerted authorities to similarities between his death and the death of Glenn Turner leading to her arrest and conviction

[89] P Ann Miller Kontz, born 1970, US, research chemist, arrested 2004, sentenced to 25 years imprisonment **2005**

PA Arsenic administered in food and drink

V Husband Eric Miller, a paediatric AIDS researcher, 2000 (Raleigh, North Carolina)

M To be with her lover Derril Willard

R Lamb (2005)

[90] P Charles Higgs, born 1964, US, critical care nurse, sentenced to life imprisonment **2007**

PA Succinylcholine chloride injection

V His wife former State Controller Kathy Augustine, 2006 (ill at her Reno, Nevada home, died three days later in Reno medical centre)

M Marital discord

R Smith (2008)

[91] P James Keown, born 1974, US, radio reporter, sentenced to life imprisonment **2008**

PA Antifreeze administered in Gatorade

V Wife Julie, a registered nurse, 2004, (Waltham, Massachusetts)

M Financial gain from life insurance

R *Hopkinton News* (2008)

N Checks of perpetrator's computer revealed searches for ethylene glycol poisoning

[92] P Stacey Castor, born 1967, New York, US, arrested 2007, sentenced to life imprisonment **2009** for second-degree murder, died 2016

PA Antifreeze apparently force fed when victim in a weak state

V David Castor, her second husband, 2005 (Onondaga County, New York)

M Financial gain from inheritance

R Associated Press 6 March 2009

N Attempted to murder her daughter Ashley Wallace in 2007 with pills mixed with vodka; suspected of murdering her first husband Michael Wallace in 2000

[93] P Lakvir Singh, born 1969, India, sentenced to life imprisonment **2010**

PA Aconite secretly added to a curry in refrigerator at Cheema's home

V Her lover Lakhvinder Cheema, 2009 (administered at his house in London, died in hospital)

M Jealousy over Cheema's plans to marry someone else

R BBC News 11 February 2010

[94] P K. D. Kempanna (Mallika), born 1965, India, sentenced to death then commuted to life imprisonment **2012**

PA Cyanide, administered in food

V Six women temple worshipers from 1999 to 2007, killed at remote temple sites where KDK had lured them

M Financial gain from robbery

R *Times of India* 24 March 2009

[95] P Paul Marshall Curry, born 1956, US, sentenced to life imprisonment without parole **2014**

PA Nicotine injection following a sedative, appears PMC poisoned the victim for a considerable period before killing her

V Wife Linda in 1995, at their home in San Clemente

M Financial gain from life insurance

R Robinson (2014)

N Police suspected murder at the time but lacked the evidence to bring charges until years later

[96] P Lacey Spears; born 1988; Alabama, US; single mother; sentenced to 20 years imprisonment for second-degree murder **2015**

PA Sodium (salt) administered through stomach feeding tube

V Her son Garnett-Paul Spears, aged 5 years; at their home in Chestnut Ridge, New York and finally in a lethal dose in hospital in New York administered through feeding tube January 2014

M Possible factitious disorder imposed on another. Possibly, final dose given when LS feared that her son would reveal she was making him ill

R Associated Press, 8 April 2015

N LS projected herself on social media as a caring mother battling with her son's mysterious complaint.

[97] P Dr. Robert Ferrante, born 1949, US, neuroscientist, sentenced to life imprisonment **2015**

PA Cyanide (bought through his laboratory) added to Creatine fertility boosting drink

V His wife Dr. Autumn Klein in 2013 (at their home in Pittsburgh)

M Feared his wife was having an affair or planning divorce, or felt pressured into having a child

R Ward (2015)

[98] P Victorino Chua, born 1966, Philippines, nurse, sentenced to 35 years imprisonment **2015**

PA Insulin injected into saline bags and ampules later unwittingly used by other nurses

V Tracey Arden 44, and Derek Weaver 83, in 2015 both patients (at hospital in Stockport, England)

M Probably sadistic

R *Manchester Evening News*, 2015; BBC News 18 May 2015

[99] P Roger Cooper, born 1974, Essex, England, Costco store manager, and David Cooper, born 1976, Essex, England, doorman, both sentenced to life imprisonment **2015**

PA Chloroform probably administered over mouth on a soaked cloth

V Sameena Imam, Roger Cooper's lover 2015 (at David Copper's home in Leicester)

M To prevent victim from revealing affair with RC

R Gibons, 21 October 2015

[100] P Jessica Wongso, born 1989, Indonesia, later resident of Australia, student, sentenced to 20 years imprisonment, **2016**

PA Cyanide in coffee at a café, Jakarta, Indonesia (died soon after in hospital)

V Friend, Wayan Salihin, aged 27 years, graphic designer, January 2016

M Jealousy over friend's success and new husband Arif Soemarko, sadism

R Topsfield (2016)

[101] P He Tiandai, born 1970, Lechang County, China; carer; sentenced to death and immediate execution, **2016**

PA Sleeping pills and dichlorvos insecticide administered in soup, then soup injected into victim's stomach and hip. As victim was dying, HT also strangled her with a piece of rope

V He Yanzhu, 70-year-old woman, Guandong Province, China (in victim's home), killed January 2015 after HT had been working for only a few days.

M Greed, family agreed if victim died before HT salary due, she would still be paid for the whole month. Possible resentment at employer's parsimony.

R Li (5 May 2016)

N HE stated that she had previously killed seven other clients.

References

Adam, H. L. (1930). *Trial of George Chapman (Notable British Trials Series)*. London: William Hodge.

Appleton, A. (1973). *Mary Ann Cotton*. London: Michael Joseph.

Associated Press. (2009, March 6). Woman Gets 50 Years in Antifreeze Murder of Husband. *New York Daily News*. 2009, 6 March. www.nydailynews.com/news/world/woman-50-years-antifreeze-murder-husband-stacy-castor-upstate-blame-daughter-article-1.366822

Associated Press. (2015, April 8). Lacy spears who killed son with salt gets leniency in sentencing. *The New York Times*. www.nytimes.com/2015/04/09/nyregion/lacey-spears-who-killed-son-with-salt-gets-leniency-in-sentencing.html?_r=0

Author Uncredited. (2004). Nurse gets life for muscle relaxant slaying. *The Japan Times*. March 31, 2004. www.japantimes.co.jp/news/2004/03/31/national/nurse-gets-life-for-muscle-relaxant-slaying

BBC News. (2010, February 11). Curry poison killer Lakhvir Singh jailed for life. http://news.bbc.co.uk/2/hi/uk_news/england/london/8509798.stm

BBC News. (2015, May 18). *Stepping Hill Nurse Victorino Chua Guilty of Murdering Patients*. www.bbc.co.uk/news/uk-england-32782153

Bennett, B. (1974). *The Noose Tightens*. Cape Town: Howard B. Timmins.

Blundell, R. H., & Seaton, R. E. (1929). *The Trial of Jean Pierre Vaquier* (Notable British Trials Series). London: William Hodge.

Boswell, C., & Thompson, L. (1961). *The Carlyle Harris Case*. New York: Collier.

Bowker, A. E. (1947). *Behind the bar*. London: Staples Press.

Browne, G. L. & Stewart, C. G. ([1883]/2015). *Reports of trials of murder by poisoning*. London: Stevens and Sons (Project Guttenberg version 2015).

Browne, D. G., & Tullett, E. V. (1951). *Sir Bernard Spilsbury: His life and cases*. London: George G. Harrap.

Buhk, T. T. (2014). *Poisoning the peck of grand rapids: The scandalous 1916 murder plot*. Charleston, SC: The History Press.

Davies, O. (2004). *'Bateman, Mary 1768-1809' Oxford Dictionary of National Biography*. Oxford: Oxford University Press.

Davy, M. (2003) Poison mystery widens after suicide note. *New York Times*. May 9, 2003. www.nytimes.com/2003/05/09/us/poison-mystery-widens-after-a-suicide-note

Dougall, C. (2016). *King, William Henry. Dictionary of Canadian Biography Vol 8 (1851–60)*. Toronto: University of Toronto.

Duke, W. (1934). *Six trials*. London: Victor Gollancz.

Emsley, J. (2005) *The elements of murder: A history of poison*. Oxford: Oxford University Press.

Fahey, J. E. (2011). The secret poison plot. Adolf Hofrichter and the Austro-Hungarian general staff. *Journal on European History of Law, 2*(1), 66–71.

Farrell, M. (1989a). Arsenic poisoning and the Armstrong case. *Solicitors Journal, 133(34)*, 1074–1075.

Farrell, M. (1989b). Many faced poison. *Police Review, 97*(5032), 2022–2023.

Farrell, M. (1990). Arsenic and the Charlotte Bryant Case. *Solicitors Journal, 134*(14), 393–394.

Farrell, M. (1992). *Poisons and poisoners: An encyclopaedia of homicidal poisonings*. London: Robert Hale.

Farrell, M. (1993a). What's your poison? *Solicitors Journal*. March 19, 1993.

Farrell, M. (1993b). Death certification and Neil Cream's murder of matilda clover. *The Criminologist, 17*(4), 237–241.

Farrell, M. (1994). The murders of Mary Wilson. *Justice of the Peace, 158*(32), 523–525.

Farrell, M. (1995). Police and poisoners. *The Police Journal, 68*(2), 168–170.

Foran, D. R., Wills, B. E., Kiley, B. M., Jackson, C. B., & Trestrail, J. H., III. (2011). The conviction of Dr. Crippen: New Forensic findings in a century old murder (Case Report Criminalistics). *Journal of Forensic Sciences, 56*(1), 233–240.

Friedland, M. L. (1984). *The trials of Isrel Lipski: a true story of a victorian murder in the east end of London*. New York: Beaufort Books.

Gibons, D. (2015, October 21).Coventry Costco murder: Brothers Jailed for thirty years after killing Sameena Imam. *Coventry telegraph* www.coventrytelegraph.net/news/coventry-news/coventry-costco-murder-brothers-jailed-10307312

Glaister, J. (1954). *The power of poison*. London: C. Johnson.

Glatt, J. (2004). *Deadly American Beauty*. New York: MacMillan (St. Martin's Press) www.legacy.sandiegouniontribune.com/news/metro/rossum/

Gorman, A. (2004). Wife get death for killing husband. *Los Angeles Times*. 2004, January 13. www.articles.latimes.com/2004/jan/13/local/me-poison13

Hanna, J. (1999) Ex-nurse gets maximum term in hospital killings. *Chicago Tribune*, 1999, November 16. http://articles.chicagotribune.com/1999-11-16/news/9911160161_1_vermillion-county-hospital-orville-lynn-majors-hospital-killings and www.law.justia.com/cases/indiana/supreme-court/2002/08140201-rts

Heppenstall, R. (1970) *French crime in the romantic age*. London: Hamish Hamilton.

Hickey, E. (2010). *Serial murderers and their victims* (5th ed.). Belmont, CA.: Wadsorth.

Holmes, P. (1968). *The trials of Dr. Copollino*. David McKay: New York.

Hoo, S. (2003) *Rat poison revenge growing in China*. (www.rense.com/general44/grow)

Hopkinton News, (2008), Keown found guilty of first degree murder in connection with poisoning death of his wife Julie. *Hopkinton News*. July 2, 2008 www.hopnews.com/justice_07_02_08.htm

Irving, H. B. (1912) *Trial of Mrs. Maybrick* (Notable English Trials Series). London: Hodge.

Kershaw, A. (1974) *Murder in France.* London: Constable.

Lamb, A. (2005). Kontz avoids life sentence with plea deal in husband's death. *WRAL*. November 8, 2005 and July 24, 2007 www.wral.com/news/local/story/121692/

Li L., Death sentence for carer. *Shanghai Daily.* May 5, 2016www.shanghaidaily.com/nation/Death-sentence-for-carer-who.../shdaily.shtml

McDonald, R. R. (1986). *Black Widow*. New York: St. Martin's Press.

Maeder, T. (1980). *The unspeakable crimes of Dr. Petiot Boston.* MA: Little Brown.

Manchester Evening News. (2015). *Stepping Hill Hospital Poison Nurse Victorino Chua Guilty of Murdering Patients.* May 19, 2015. www.manchestereveningnews.co.uk/news/greater-manchester-news/chua-guilty-stepping-hill-poison-9193357

Martinez, E. (2010) Antifreeze Killer Lynn turner dies in prison. *CBS News*. August 31, 2010 www.cbsnews.com/news/antifreeze-killer-lynn-turner-dies-in-prison

Morikawa, T. (1977). *The truth about the Teigin Incident.* Tokyo: Kodansha.

Nash, J. R. (1981). *Look for the woman: A narrative encyclopaedia of female poisoners, kidnappers, thieves, extrotionists, terrorists, swindlers, and spies from Elizabethan Times to the present day*. New York: M. Evans.

New York Times. (1884, May 11) *Marie Jeanneret's Death-Grim facts in the career of this famous poisoner* (p. 5). Reprinted from *The London Daily News.*

Oddie, S. I. (1941) *Inquest.* London: Hutchinson.

Parry, L. (1927). *Some famous medical trials*. London, Churchill.

Peters, C. (2005/2006). *Harold Shipman: Mind set on murder–Why Shipman killed and killed again–The true story.* London: André Deutsch.

Phelps, W. H. (2010). *The Devil's rooming house: The true story of America's deadliest serial killer*. Guilford, CN: Lyons Press.

Quotidien Le Gaulois. (1874, September 11). *Moreau – L'Herboriste de Saint-Denis* (Source: gallica.bnf.fr).

Read, S. (2005) *On the house: The Bizarre killing of Michael Malloy*. New York: Berkley Publishing.

Robinson, W. (2014) *Husband sentenced to life in prison for poisoning his wife 20 years ago with fatal nicotine dose so he could collect her $500,000 life insurance*. Mail on Line and Associated Press. 2014, November 14 and 15. http://www.dailymail.co.uk/news/article-2835347/Man-sentenced-life-fatal-nicotine-poisoning.html

Rodell, M. F. (Ed.). (1947). *San Francisco Murders*. Sloan and Pearce: New York, Duell.

Roueche, B. (1982). Annals of medicine—The prognosis for this patient is horrible. *The New Yorker* (pp. 57–71). January 25, 1982.

Roughhead, W. (Ed.). (1906). *Trial of Dr.* William Hodge: Pritchard Edinburgh.

Rowland, J. (1957). *Criminal files* London, Arco.

Skehan, P. (date unknown). Western Australia Police Historical Society.

Smith, A. D. (Ed.) (1906). *The trial of Eugène Marie Chantrelle Notable Scottish trials series* Glasgow: William Hodge.

Smith, C. (2008). *Poisoned love: The true story of ER Nurse Chaz Higgs, his ambitious wife, and shocking murder* . New York: St. Martin's True Crime.

Smith, E. H. (1923). *Famous American poison mysteries*. London: Hurst and Blackett. https://babel.hathitrust.org/cgi/pt?id=mdp.39015002619321;view=1up;seq=15

St. Aubyn, G. (1971). *Infamous victorians: Lamson and Palmer, two notorious poisoners*. London: Faber and Faber.

Stewart, J. B. (1999). *Blind eye: How the medical establishment let a Doctor get away with murder*. New York: Simon and Schuster.

Tallant, R. (1953). *Murder in New Orleans*. London: William Kimber.

Thorwald, J. (1966). *Proof of poison*. London: Thames and Hudson (Translated from the German by Richard and Clara Wilson).

Times of India. March 24, 2009. www.timesofindia.indiatimes.com/india/Woman-serial... Cyanide-Mallika.../4311321.cm

Topsfield, J. (2016). Cyanide coffee murder: Australian resident Jessica Wongso jailed for 20 years. *The Sydney Morning Herald.* October 28, 2015.

Trestrail, J. H. (2007).*Criminal poisoning: Investigational guide for law enforcement, toxicologists, forensic scientists and attorneys.* Totowa, NJ: Humana Press.

Ward, P. R. (2015). Ferrante sentenced to life in cyanide poisoning death of wife Autumn Klein. *Pittsburgh Post-Gazette.*

Washington Times. (2015). Blanche Moore. www.washingtontimes.com/news/2015/dec/20/blanche-taylor-moore-remains-on-death-row-after-25/

Watson, E. R. (Ed.). ([1856]/1952). *Trial of William Palmer (Notable British Trials Series)* ((3rd ed.) London: William Hodge.

Whittington-Egan, M. (2012). *Murder on the bluff: The carew poisoning case Glasgow.* Scotland: Neil Wilson Publishing.

Wilson, C., & Seaman, D. (1983). *Encyclopedia of modern murder: 1962–1982.* London: Barker.

Wilson, P. (1971). *Murderess* London: Michael Joseph.

Young, F. (Ed.) (1927). *The trial of Herbert Rowse Armstrong* (Notable British Trials Series). Edinburgh: William Hodge.

Young, F. (Ed.). (1950). *The Trial of Hawley Harvey Crippen* (2nd ed.). (Notable British Trials Series). London: William Hodge. https://archive.org/stream/trialofhawleyhar00cripiala/trialofhawleyhar00cripiala_djvu.txt

Young, F. (Ed.) ([1914]/1952). *Trial of the seddons* (Notable British Trials Series). London: William Hodge.

Index

M. Farrell, *Criminology of Homicidal Poisoning*,
DOI 10.1007/978-3-319-59117-9

MIX
Papier aus verantwortungsvollen Quellen
Paper from responsible sources
FSC® C105338

If you have any concerns about our products,
you can contact us on
ProductSafety@springernature.com

In case Publisher is established outside the EU,
the EU authorized representative is:
Springer Nature Customer Service Center GmbH
Europaplatz 3, 69115 Heidelberg, Germany

Printed by Libri Plureos GmbH
in Hamburg, Germany